EMR First Responder Exam

SECRETS

Study Guide
Your Key to Exam Success

EMR Test Review for the
NREMT Emergency Medical
Responder Exam

Dear Future Exam Success Story:

First of all, **THANK YOU** for purchasing Mometrix study materials!

Second, congratulations! You are one of the few determined test-takers who are committed to doing whatever it takes to excel on your exam. **You have come to the right place.** We developed these study materials with one goal in mind: to deliver you the information you need in a format that's concise and easy to use.

In addition to optimizing your guide for the content of the test, we've outlined our recommended steps for breaking down the preparation process into small, attainable goals so you can make sure you stay on track.

We've also analyzed the entire test-taking process, identifying the most common pitfalls and showing how you can overcome them and be ready for any curveball the test throws you.

Standardized testing is one of the biggest obstacles on your road to success, which only increases the importance of doing well in the high-pressure, high-stakes environment of test day. Your results on this test could have a significant impact on your future, and this guide provides the information and practical advice to help you achieve your full potential on test day.

Your success is our success

We would love to hear from you! If you would like to share the story of your exam success or if you have any questions or comments in regard to our products, please contact us at **800-673-8175** or **support@mometrix.com**.

Thanks again for your business and we wish you continued success!

Sincerely,
The Mometrix Test Preparation Team

Need more help? Check out our flashcards at: http://MometrixFlashcards.com/EMT

TABLE OF CONTENTS

INTRODUCTION 1

SECRET KEY #1 – PLAN BIG, STUDY SMALL 2
    INFORMATION ORGANIZATION 2
    TIME MANAGEMENT 2
    STUDY ENVIRONMENT 2

SECRET KEY #2 – MAKE YOUR STUDYING COUNT 3
    RETENTION 3
    MODALITY 3

SECRET KEY #3 – PRACTICE THE RIGHT WAY 4
    PRACTICE TEST STRATEGY 5

SECRET KEY #4 – PACE YOURSELF 6

SECRET KEY #5 – HAVE A PLAN FOR GUESSING 7
    WHEN TO START THE GUESSING PROCESS 7
    HOW TO NARROW DOWN THE CHOICES 8
    WHICH ANSWER TO CHOOSE 9

TEST-TAKING STRATEGIES 10
    QUESTION STRATEGIES 10
    ANSWER CHOICE STRATEGIES 11
    GENERAL STRATEGIES 12
    FINAL NOTES 13

PREPARATORY 15

ANATOMY AND PHYSIOLOGY 32

MEDICAL TERMINOLOGY 33

PATHOPHYSIOLOGY 34

LIFE SPAN DEVELOPMENT 35

PUBLIC HEALTH 36

AIRWAY MANAGEMENT, RESPIRATIONS AND ARTIFICIAL VENTILATION 37

ASSESSMENT 43

MEDICINE 45

SHOCK AND RESUSCITATION 57

TRAUMA 60

SPECIAL PATIENT POPULATIONS 68

EMS OPERATIONS 75

EMR PRACTICE TEST 92

ANSWER KEY AND EXPLANATIONS 105

HOW TO OVERCOME TEST ANXIETY 115
    CAUSES OF TEST ANXIETY 115
    ELEMENTS OF TEST ANXIETY 116

EFFECTS OF TEST ANXIETY 116
PHYSICAL STEPS FOR BEATING TEST ANXIETY 117
MENTAL STEPS FOR BEATING TEST ANXIETY 118
STUDY STRATEGY 119
TEST TIPS 121
IMPORTANT QUALIFICATION 122

THANK YOU **123**

ADDITIONAL BONUS MATERIAL **124**

Introduction

Thank you for purchasing this resource! You have made the choice to prepare yourself for a test that could have a huge impact on your future, and this guide is designed to help you be fully ready for test day. Obviously, it's important to have a solid understanding of the test material, but you also need to be prepared for the unique environment and stressors of the test, so that you can perform to the best of your abilities.

For this purpose, the first section that appears in this guide is the **Secret Keys**. We've devoted countless hours to meticulously researching what works and what doesn't, and we've boiled down our findings to the five most impactful steps you can take to improve your performance on the test. We start at the beginning with study planning and move through the preparation process, all the way to the testing strategies that will help you get the most out of what you know when you're finally sitting in front of the test.

We recommend that you start preparing for your test as far in advance as possible. However, if you've bought this guide as a last-minute study resource and only have a few days before your test, we recommend that you skip over the first two Secret Keys since they address a long-term study plan.

If you struggle with **test anxiety**, we strongly encourage you to check out our recommendations for how you can overcome it. Test anxiety is a formidable foe, but it can be beaten, and we want to make sure you have the tools you need to defeat it.

Secret Key #1 – Plan Big, Study Small

There's a lot riding on your performance. If you want to ace this test, you're going to need to keep your skills sharp and the material fresh in your mind. You need a plan that lets you review everything you need to know while still fitting in your schedule. We'll break this strategy down into three categories.

Information Organization

Start with the information you already have: the official test outline. From this, you can make a complete list of all the concepts you need to cover before the test. Organize these concepts into groups that can be studied together, and create a list of any related vocabulary you need to learn so you can brush up on any difficult terms. You'll want to keep this vocabulary list handy once you actually start studying since you may need to add to it along the way.

Time Management

Once you have your set of study concepts, decide how to spread them out over the time you have left before the test. Break your study plan into small, clear goals so you have a manageable task for each day and know exactly what you're doing. Then just focus on one small step at a time. When you manage your time this way, you don't need to spend hours at a time studying. Studying a small block of content for a short period each day helps you retain information better and avoid stressing over how much you have left to do. You can relax knowing that you have a plan to cover everything in time. In order for this strategy to be effective though, you have to start studying early and stick to your schedule. Avoid the exhaustion and futility that comes from last-minute cramming!

Study Environment

The environment you study in has a big impact on your learning. Studying in a coffee shop, while probably more enjoyable, is not likely to be as fruitful as studying in a quiet room. It's important to keep distractions to a minimum. You're only planning to study for a short block of time, so make the most of it. Don't pause to check your phone or get up to find a snack. It's also important to **avoid multitasking**. Research has consistently shown that multitasking will make your studying dramatically less effective. Your study area should also be comfortable and well-lit so you don't have the distraction of straining your eyes or sitting on an uncomfortable chair.

The time of day you study is also important. You want to be rested and alert. Don't wait until just before bedtime. Study when you'll be most likely to comprehend and remember. Even better, if you know what time of day your test will be, set that time aside for study. That way your brain will be used to working on that subject at that specific time and you'll have a better chance of recalling information.

Finally, it can be helpful to team up with others who are studying for the same test. Your actual studying should be done in as isolated an environment as possible, but the work of organizing the information and setting up the study plan can be divided up. In between study sessions, you can discuss with your teammates the concepts that you're all studying and quiz each other on the details. Just be sure that your teammates are as serious about the test as you are. If you find that your study time is being replaced with social time, you might need to find a new team.

Secret Key #2 – Make Your Studying Count

You're devoting a lot of time and effort to preparing for this test, so you want to be absolutely certain it will pay off. This means doing more than just reading the content and hoping you can remember it on test day. It's important to make every minute of study count. There are two main areas you can focus on to make your studying count:

Retention

It doesn't matter how much time you study if you can't remember the material. You need to make sure you are retaining the concepts. To check your retention of the information you're learning, try recalling it at later times with minimal prompting. Try carrying around flashcards and glance at one or two from time to time or ask a friend who's also studying for the test to quiz you.

To enhance your retention, look for ways to put the information into practice so that you can apply it rather than simply recalling it. If you're using the information in practical ways, it will be much easier to remember. Similarly, it helps to solidify a concept in your mind if you're not only reading it to yourself but also explaining it to someone else. Ask a friend to let you teach them about a concept you're a little shaky on (or speak aloud to an imaginary audience if necessary). As you try to summarize, define, give examples, and answer your friend's questions, you'll understand the concepts better and they will stay with you longer. Finally, step back for a big picture view and ask yourself how each piece of information fits with the whole subject. When you link the different concepts together and see them working together as a whole, it's easier to remember the individual components.

Finally, practice showing your work on any multi-step problems, even if you're just studying. Writing out each step you take to solve a problem will help solidify the process in your mind, and you'll be more likely to remember it during the test.

Modality

Modality simply refers to the means or method by which you study. Choosing a study modality that fits your own individual learning style is crucial. No two people learn best in exactly the same way, so it's important to know your strengths and use them to your advantage.

For example, if you learn best by visualization, focus on visualizing a concept in your mind and draw an image or a diagram. Try color-coding your notes, illustrating them, or creating symbols that will trigger your mind to recall a learned concept. If you learn best by hearing or discussing information, find a study partner who learns the same way or read aloud to yourself. Think about how to put the information in your own words. Imagine that you are giving a lecture on the topic and record yourself so you can listen to it later.

For any learning style, flashcards can be helpful. Organize the information so you can take advantage of spare moments to review. Underline key words or phrases. Use different colors for different categories. Mnemonic devices (such as creating a short list in which every item starts with the same letter) can also help with retention. Find what works best for you and use it to store the information in your mind most effectively and easily.

Secret Key #3 – Practice the Right Way

Your success on test day depends not only on how many hours you put into preparing, but also on whether you prepared the right way. It's good to check along the way to see if your studying is paying off. One of the most effective ways to do this is by taking practice tests to evaluate your progress. Practice tests are useful because they show exactly where you need to improve. Every time you take a practice test, pay special attention to these three groups of questions:

- The questions you got wrong
- The questions you had to guess on, even if you guessed right
- The questions you found difficult or slow to work through

This will show you exactly what your weak areas are, and where you need to devote more study time. Ask yourself why each of these questions gave you trouble. Was it because you didn't understand the material? Was it because you didn't remember the vocabulary? Do you need more repetitions on this type of question to build speed and confidence? Dig into those questions and figure out how you can strengthen your weak areas as you go back to review the material.

Additionally, many practice tests have a section explaining the answer choices. It can be tempting to read the explanation and think that you now have a good understanding of the concept. However, an explanation likely only covers part of the question's broader context. Even if the explanation makes sense, **go back and investigate** every concept related to the question until you're positive you have a thorough understanding.

As you go along, keep in mind that the practice test is just that: practice. Memorizing these questions and answers will not be very helpful on the actual test because it is unlikely to have any of the same exact questions. If you only know the right answers to the sample questions, you won't be prepared for the real thing. **Study the concepts** until you understand them fully, and then you'll be able to answer any question that shows up on the test.

It's important to wait on the practice tests until you're ready. If you take a test on your first day of study, you may be overwhelmed by the amount of material covered and how much you need to learn. Work up to it gradually.

On test day, you'll need to be prepared for answering questions, managing your time, and using the test-taking strategies you've learned. It's a lot to balance, like a mental marathon that will have a big impact on your future. Like training for a marathon, you'll need to start slowly and work your way up. When test day arrives, you'll be ready.

Start with the strategies you've read in the first two Secret Keys—plan your course and study in the way that works best for you. If you have time, consider using multiple study resources to get different approaches to the same concepts. It can be helpful to see difficult concepts from more than one angle. Then find a good source for practice tests. Many times, the test website will suggest potential study resources or provide sample tests.

Practice Test Strategy

When you're ready to start taking practice tests, follow this strategy:

1. Take the first test with no time constraints and with your notes and study guide handy. Take your time and focus on applying the strategies you've learned.
2. Take the second practice test open-book as well, but set a timer and practice pacing yourself to finish in time.
3. Take any other practice tests as if it were test day. Set a timer and put away your study materials. Sit at a table or desk in a quiet room, imagine yourself at the testing center, and answer questions as quickly and accurately as possible.
4. Keep repeating step 3 on a regular basis until you run out of practice tests or it's time for the actual test. Your mind will be ready for the schedule and stress of test day, and you'll be able to focus on recalling the material you've learned.

Secret Key #4 – Pace Yourself

Once you're fully prepared for the material on the test, your biggest challenge on test day will be managing your time. Just knowing that the clock is ticking can make you panic even if you have plenty of time left. Work on pacing yourself so you can build confidence against the time constraints of the exam. Pacing is a difficult skill to master, especially in a high-pressure environment, so **practice is vital**.

Set time expectations for your pace based on how much time is available. For example, if a section has 60 questions and the time limit is 30 minutes, you know you have to average 30 seconds or less per question in order to answer them all. Although 30 seconds is the hard limit, set 25 seconds per question as your goal, so you reserve extra time to spend on harder questions. When you budget extra time for the harder questions, you no longer have any reason to stress when those questions take longer to answer.

Don't let this time expectation distract you from working through the test at a calm, steady pace, but keep it in mind so you don't spend too much time on any one question. Recognize that taking extra time on one question you don't understand may keep you from answering two that you do understand later in the test. If your time limit for a question is up and you're still not sure of the answer, mark it and move on, and come back to it later if the time and the test format allow. If the testing format doesn't allow you to return to earlier questions, just make an educated guess; then put it out of your mind and move on.

On the easier questions, be careful not to rush. It may seem wise to hurry through them so you have more time for the challenging ones, but it's not worth missing one if you know the concept and just didn't take the time to read the question fully. Work efficiently but make sure you understand the question and have looked at all of the answer choices, since more than one may seem right at first.

Even if you're paying attention to the time, you may find yourself a little behind at some point. You should speed up to get back on track, but do so wisely. Don't panic; just take a few seconds less on each question until you're caught up. Don't guess without thinking, but do look through the answer choices and eliminate any you know are wrong. If you can get down to two choices, it is often worthwhile to guess from those. Once you've chosen an answer, move on and don't dwell on any that you skipped or had to hurry through. If a question was taking too long, chances are it was one of the harder ones, so you weren't as likely to get it right anyway.

On the other hand, if you find yourself getting ahead of schedule, it may be beneficial to slow down a little. The more quickly you work, the more likely you are to make a careless mistake that will affect your score. You've budgeted time for each question, so don't be afraid to spend that time. Practice an efficient but careful pace to get the most out of the time you have.

Secret Key #5 – Have a Plan for Guessing

When you're taking the test, you may find yourself stuck on a question. Some of the answer choices seem better than others, but you don't see the one answer choice that is obviously correct. What do you do?

The scenario described above is very common, yet most test takers have not effectively prepared for it. Developing and practicing a plan for guessing may be one of the single most effective uses of your time as you get ready for the exam.

In developing your plan for guessing, there are three questions to address:

- When should you start the guessing process?
- How should you narrow down the choices?
- Which answer should you choose?

When to Start the Guessing Process

Unless your plan for guessing is to select C every time (which, despite its merits, is not what we recommend), you need to leave yourself enough time to apply your answer elimination strategies. Since you have a limited amount of time for each question, that means that if you're going to give yourself the best shot at guessing correctly, you have to decide quickly whether or not you will guess.

Of course, the best-case scenario is that you don't have to guess at all, so first, see if you can answer the question based on your knowledge of the subject and basic reasoning skills. Focus on the key words in the question and try to jog your memory of related topics. Give yourself a chance to bring the knowledge to mind, but once you realize that you don't have (or you can't access) the knowledge you need to answer the question, it's time to start the guessing process.

It's almost always better to start the guessing process too early than too late. It only takes a few seconds to remember something and answer the question from knowledge. Carefully eliminating wrong answer choices takes longer. Plus, going through the process of eliminating answer choices can actually help jog your memory.

Summary: Start the guessing process as soon as you decide that you can't answer the question based on your knowledge.

How to Narrow Down the Choices

The next chapter in this book (**Test-Taking Strategies**) includes a wide range of strategies for how to approach questions and how to look for answer choices to eliminate. You will definitely want to read those carefully, practice them, and figure out which ones work best for you. Here though, we're going to address a mindset rather than a particular strategy.

Your chances of guessing an answer correctly depend on how many options you are choosing from.

How many choices you have	How likely you are to guess correctly
5	20%
4	25%
3	33%
2	50%
1	100%

You can see from this chart just how valuable it is to be able to eliminate incorrect answers and make an educated guess, but there are two things that many test takers do that cause them to miss out on the benefits of guessing:

- Accidentally eliminating the correct answer
- Selecting an answer based on an impression

We'll look at the first one here, and the second one in the next section.

To avoid accidentally eliminating the correct answer, we recommend a thought exercise called **the $5 challenge**. In this challenge, you only eliminate an answer choice from contention if you are willing to bet $5 on it being wrong. Why $5? Five dollars is a small but not insignificant amount of money. It's an amount you could afford to lose but wouldn't want to throw away. And while losing $5 once might not hurt too much, doing it twenty times will set you back $100. In the same way, each small decision you make—eliminating a choice here, guessing on a question there—won't by itself impact your score very much, but when you put them all together, they can make a big difference. By holding each answer choice elimination decision to a higher standard, you can reduce the risk of accidentally eliminating the correct answer.

The $5 challenge can also be applied in a positive sense: If you are willing to bet $5 that an answer choice *is* correct, go ahead and mark it as correct.

Summary: Only eliminate an answer choice if you are willing to bet $5 that it is wrong.

Which Answer to Choose

You're taking the test. You've run into a hard question and decided you'll have to guess. You've eliminated all the answer choices you're willing to bet $5 on. Now you have to pick an answer. Why do we even need to talk about this? Why can't you just pick whichever one you feel like when the time comes?

The answer to these questions is that if you don't come into the test with a plan, you'll rely on your impression to select an answer choice, and if you do that, you risk falling into a trap. The test writers know that everyone who takes their test will be guessing on some of the questions, so they intentionally write wrong answer choices to seem plausible. You still have to pick an answer though, and if the wrong answer choices are designed to look right, how can you ever be sure that you're not falling for their trap? The best solution we've found to this dilemma is to take the decision out of your hands entirely. Here is the process we recommend:

Once you've eliminated any choices that you are confident (willing to bet $5) are wrong, select the first remaining choice as your answer.

Whether you choose to select the first remaining choice, the second, or the last, the important thing is that you use some preselected standard. Using this approach guarantees that you will not be enticed into selecting an answer choice that looks right, because you are not basing your decision on how the answer choices look.

This is not meant to make you question your knowledge. Instead, it is to help you recognize the difference between your knowledge and your impressions. There's a huge difference between thinking an answer is right because of what you know, and thinking an answer is right because it looks or sounds like it should be right.

Summary: To ensure that your selection is appropriately random, make a predetermined selection from among all answer choices you have not eliminated.

Test-Taking Strategies

This section contains a list of test-taking strategies that you may find helpful as you work through the test. By taking what you know and applying logical thought, you can maximize your chances of answering any question correctly!

It is very important to realize that every question is different and every person is different: no single strategy will work on every question, and no single strategy will work for every person. That's why we've included all of them here, so you can try them out and determine which ones work best for different types of questions and which ones work best for you.

Question Strategies

Read Carefully

Read the question and answer choices carefully. Don't miss the question because you misread the terms. You have plenty of time to read each question thoroughly and make sure you understand what is being asked. Yet a happy medium must be attained, so don't waste too much time. You must read carefully, but efficiently.

Contextual Clues

Look for contextual clues. If the question includes a word you are not familiar with, look at the immediate context for some indication of what the word might mean. Contextual clues can often give you all the information you need to decipher the meaning of an unfamiliar word. Even if you can't determine the meaning, you may be able to narrow down the possibilities enough to make a solid guess at the answer to the question.

Prefixes

If you're having trouble with a word in the question or answer choices, try dissecting it. Take advantage of every clue that the word might include. Prefixes and suffixes can be a huge help. Usually they allow you to determine a basic meaning. Pre- means before, post- means after, pro - is positive, de- is negative. From prefixes and suffixes, you can get an idea of the general meaning of the word and try to put it into context.

Hedge Words

Watch out for critical hedge words, such as *likely, may, can, sometimes, often, almost, mostly, usually, generally, rarely*, and *sometimes*. Question writers insert these hedge phrases to cover every possibility. Often an answer choice will be wrong simply because it leaves no room for exception. Be on guard for answer choices that have definitive words such as *exactly* and *always*.

Switchback Words

Stay alert for *switchbacks*. These are the words and phrases frequently used to alert you to shifts in thought. The most common switchback words are *but, although*, and *however*. Others include *nevertheless, on the other hand, even though, while, in spite of, despite, regardless of*. Switchback words are important to catch because they can change the direction of the question or an answer choice.

Face Value

When in doubt, use common sense. Accept the situation in the problem at face value. Don't read too much into it. These problems will not require you to make wild assumptions. If you have to go beyond creativity and warp time or space in order to have an answer choice fit the question, then you should move on and consider the other answer choices. These are normal problems rooted in reality. The applicable relationship or explanation may not be readily apparent, but it is there for you to figure out. Use your common sense to interpret anything that isn't clear.

Answer Choice Strategies

Answer Selection

The most thorough way to pick an answer choice is to identify and eliminate wrong answers until only one is left, then confirm it is the correct answer. Sometimes an answer choice may immediately seem right, but be careful. The test writers will usually put more than one reasonable answer choice on each question, so take a second to read all of them and make sure that the other choices are not equally obvious. As long as you have time left, it is better to read every answer choice than to pick the first one that looks right without checking the others.

Eliminate Answers

Eliminate answer choices as soon as you realize they are wrong, but make sure you consider all possibilities. If you are eliminating answer choices and realize that the last one you are left with is also wrong, don't panic. Start over and consider each choice again. There may be something you missed the first time that you will realize on the second pass.

Avoid Fact Traps

Don't be distracted by an answer choice that is factually true but doesn't answer the question. You are looking for the choice that answers the question. Stay focused on what the question is asking for so you don't accidentally pick an answer that is true but incorrect. Always go back to the question and make sure the answer choice you've selected actually answers the question and is not merely a true statement.

Extreme Statements

In general, you should avoid answers that put forth extreme actions as standard practice or proclaim controversial ideas as established fact. An answer choice that states the "process should be used in certain situations, if..." is much more likely to be correct than one that states the "process should be discontinued completely." The first is a calm rational statement and doesn't even make a definitive, uncompromising stance, using a hedge word *if* to provide wiggle room, whereas the second choice is a radical idea and far more extreme.

Benchmark

As you read through the answer choices and you come across one that seems to answer the question well, mentally select that answer choice. This is not your final answer, but it's the one that will help you evaluate the other answer choices. The one that you selected is your benchmark or standard for judging each of the other answer choices. Every other answer choice must be compared to your benchmark. That choice is correct until proven otherwise by another answer choice beating it. If you find a better answer, then that one becomes your new benchmark. Once

- 11 -

you've decided that no other choice answers the question as well as your benchmark, you have your final answer.

Predict the Answer

Before you even start looking at the answer choices, it is often best to try to predict the answer. When you come up with the answer on your own, it is easier to avoid distractions and traps because you will know exactly what to look for. The right answer choice is unlikely to be word-for-word what you came up with, but it should be a close match. Even if you are confident that you have the right answer, you should still take the time to read each option before moving on.

General Strategies

Tough Questions

If you are stumped on a problem or it appears too hard or too difficult, don't waste time. Move on! Remember though, if you can quickly check for obviously incorrect answer choices, your chances of guessing correctly are greatly improved. Before you completely give up, at least try to knock out a couple of possible answers. Eliminate what you can and then guess at the remaining answer choices before moving on.

Check Your Work

Since you will probably not know every term listed and the answer to every question, it is important that you get credit for the ones that you do know. Don't miss any questions through careless mistakes. If at all possible, try to take a second to look back over your answer selection and make sure you've selected the correct answer choice and haven't made a costly careless mistake (such as marking an answer choice that you didn't mean to mark). This quick double check should more than pay for itself in caught mistakes for the time it costs.

Pace Yourself

It's easy to be overwhelmed when you're looking at a page full of questions; your mind is confused and full of random thoughts, and the clock is ticking down faster than you would like. Calm down and maintain the pace that you have set for yourself. Especially as you get down to the last few minutes of the test, don't let the small numbers on the clock make you panic. As long as you are on track by monitoring your pace, you are guaranteed to have time for each question.

Don't Rush

It is very easy to make errors when you are in a hurry. Maintaining a fast pace in answering questions is pointless if it makes you miss questions that you would have gotten right otherwise. Test writers like to include distracting information and wrong answers that seem right. Taking a little extra time to avoid careless mistakes can make all the difference in your test score. Find a pace that allows you to be confident in the answers that you select.

Keep Moving

Panicking will not help you pass the test, so do your best to stay calm and keep moving. Taking deep breaths and going through the answer elimination steps you practiced can help to break through a stress barrier and keep your pace.

Final Notes

The combination of a solid foundation of content knowledge and the confidence that comes from practicing your plan for applying that knowledge is the key to maximizing your performance on test day. As your foundation of content knowledge is built up and strengthened, you'll find that the strategies included in this chapter become more and more effective in helping you quickly sift through the distractions and traps of the test to isolate the correct answer.

Now it's time to move on to the test content chapters of this book, but be sure to keep your goal in mind. As you read, think about how you will be able to apply this information on the test. If you've already seen sample questions for the test and you have an idea of the question format and style, try to come up with questions of your own that you can answer based on what you're reading. This will give you valuable practice applying your knowledge in the same ways you can expect to on test day.

Good luck and good studying!

Preparatory

EMS systems

The National Highway Traffic Safety Administration is the lead agency for coordinating and promoting evidence-based emergency medical services (EMS) (fire based, third service, and hospital based) and the 9-1-1 system. The public-safety answering point (PSAP) is the designated call-receiving site that directs calls to the appropriate emergency services. Each state defines the scope of practice, licensure, and credentialing for prehospital personnel and sets education standards based on national EMS standards. The emergency medical responder (EMR) is expected to maintain certification through maintenance of skills and continuing education and should exhibit professional behavior, including working with integrity and empathy, being an effective member of a team, showing respect and tact, maintaining a professional appearance, communicating effectively, and advocating for patients. The EMR must be alert to patient safety and recognize that most errors result from skills-based, rules-based, and knowledge-based failures. Error reduction requires the use of decision aids and protocols, asking for assistance when appropriate, questioning assumptions, and debriefing calls.

National EMS Education Agenda for the Future: A Systems Approach

The **National EMS Education Agenda for the Future: A Systems Approach** proposed an education system for EMS with five primary components, establishing the following goals for 2010 and 2020:

1. Core content: Core content to be developed by the EMS medical community, educators, and providers under the leadership of the National Highway Traffic Safety Administration (NHTSA) to ensure consistency of content and reciprocity of certification. The core content should be tied to licensure and accreditation.
2. Scope-of-practice model: National models to be used by states for all levels of EMS certification/licensure.
3. Education standards: Standards developed by EMS educators with input from the medical community and regulators that are peer reviewed.
4. Education program accreditation: A single national accreditation agency will develop standards and guidelines.
5. EMS certification: Four levels of national certification with different educational requirements, standards, scopes of practice, and certification: (1) entry-level emergency medical responder (EMR), (2) next-level emergency medical technician (EMT), (3) advanced EMT (AEMT), and (4) paramedic.

Roles and responsibilities of EMS personnel

Roles and responsibilities of EMS personnel include the following:

- Maintain the readiness of all equipment, including disinfecting, packaging, and storing.
- Monitor personal safety, patient safety, and the safety of others on the scene.
- Evaluate the scene for additional resources when indicated.
- Gain access to the patient only when it is safe to do so.
- Perform an assessment of the patient's condition and needs.
- Provide emergency medical care as needed (or until additional resources arrive).
- Provide emotional support to the patient, family, and other providers.

- 15 -

- Maintain the continuity of care.
- Ensure that medical and legal standards are upheld and that patient privacy is protected.
- Communicate with others and maintain community relations.
- Practice professional behavior (integrity, self-motivation, self-confidence, tact, respect, and professional appearance).
- Maintain certification and meet continuing education requirements.

Patient safety and high-risk situations

Patients are especially at risk of further injury or death in high-risk situations and activities such as the following:

- Hand-off: A standard procedure such as SBAR should be used, as follows:
    - (S) = Situation: Overview of current situation and important issues.
    - (B) = Background: Important history and issues leading to current situation.
    - (A) = Assessment: Summary of important facts and condition.
    - (R) = Recommendation: Actions needed.

- Communications: Problems may result in delayed or inadequate care, wrong address, or wrong destination.
- Dropping: Patients can be easily dropped if the gurney isn't positioned properly or if too few personnel are involved in transport.
- Ambulance crashes: Unnecessary speeding and failing to stop at intersections are the most common causes of ambulance crashes.
- Inadequate spinal immobilization: If unsure, it's always best to immobilize.

Quality improvement

Quality improvement requires that an organization or system continually evaluates processes and outcomes and takes measures to improve the quality of care. The focus of quality improvement is on patient safety in access, provision of care, transport, and hand-off. Errors are often related to these different types of failures:

- Skills-based: Includes slips and mistakes. Slips occur when the EMR has the correct intent but does not carry out an action as intended, such as mistakenly using the wrong piece of equipment. Mistakes occur when the EMR has an incorrect intention that leads to incorrect action.
- Rules-based: The EMR incorrectly applies a rule, applies a bad or wrong rule, or fails to apply the correct rules. For example, an EMR is injured because of failing to assess safety before approaching a patient.
- Knowledge-based: The EMR's knowledge is not adequate for the situation.

EMS personnel can help reduce errors by debriefing, constantly reevaluating and questioning assumptions, using established protocols and decision aids, and asking for assistance when needed.

Research

Research is especially important in identifying the need for changes in procedures and protocols in order to improve patient outcomes. Research depends on the gathering of data. Data collection may include direct observations, surveys, interviews, and various other sources of information, such as documents and audiovisual materials. <u>Literature research</u> requires a comprehensive evaluation of

- 16 -

current (≤5 years) and/or historical information. Most literature research begins with an Internet search of databases, which provides listings of books, journals, and other materials on specific topics. Databases vary in content, and many contain only a reference listing with or without an abstract, so once the listing is obtained, the researcher must do a further search (publisher, library, etc.) to locate the material. Some databases require a subscription, but access is often available through educational or healthcare institutions. In order to search effectively, the researcher should begin by writing a brief explanation of the research to help identify possible keywords and synonyms to use as search words.

Data collection

When developing **data collection procedures** to determine needs, the following must be considered: the purpose of the data collection, the audience for which the data are intended, the types of questions to be answered, the scope of the research, and the resources available to carry out data collection.

Method	Issues regarding procedures
Direct observation	Observers must be selected and trained on how to observe and when and how to record observations.
Interviews	Interview questions must be developed and validated, and the interviewers must be given practice time.
Questionnaires	The type of questionnaire, the questions, and the Likert scale must be determined as well as the method of distribution (one-on-one, group, email, Internet).
Record review	A form or checklist should be developed to guide record review, and the records should be selected based on criteria established for the research.
Secondary analysis	The databases to be mined should be selected, and the criteria for the research should be established, including keywords, time frames, and populations.

Recommended immunizations for EMS personnel

The Centers for Disease Control and Prevention (CDC) recommends the following **immunizations** for all healthcare workers, including EMS personnel:

- Hepatitis B: Three-dose series (now, in one month, and five months later) followed by an anti-HBs serologic test 30 to 60 days after the third immunization.
- Measles, mumps, rubella (MMR): Two-dose series with the second immunization at least 28 days after the first for those born during or after 1957 and those born before 1957 without proof of immunity.
- Varicella (chickenpox): Two doses, four weeks apart. (A combined MMRV immunization is available.)
- Influenza: Annually.
- Tetanus, diphtheria, and pertussis (Tdap): One time with a tetanus (TD) booster every 10 years. The TD injection does not protect against pertussis (whooping cough).
- Meningococcal: One dose.

Screening for tuberculosis with a chest x-ray or skin test is also recommended.

CDC isolation guidelines

The **2007 CDC Guideline for Isolation Precautions** includes the standard precautions that apply to all patients and transmission-based precautions for those with known or suspected infections. **Standard precautions** should be used for all patients because all body fluids (sweat, urine, feces, blood, and sputum) and nonintact skin and mucous membranes may be infected.

Hand hygiene	Wash hands before and after each patient contact and after any contact with body fluids and contaminated items. Use soap and water for visible soiling.
Protective equipment	Use personal protective equipment (PPE), such as gloves, gowns, and masks, eye protection, and/or face shields, when anticipating contact with body fluids or contaminated skin.
Respiratory hygiene/ Cough etiquette	Use source-control measures, such as covering cough, disposing of tissues, using a surgical mask on the person coughing or on staff to prevent inhalation of droplets, and properly disposing of dressings and used equipment. Wash hands after contacting respiratory secretions. Maintain a distance of >3 feet from a coughing person when possible.
Sharps	Dispose of sharps, such as needles, carefully in sharps containers. Do not recap needles.

The **2007 CDC Guideline for Isolation Precautions** includes the standard precautions that apply to all patients and **transmission-based precautions** for those with known or suspected infections as well as those with excessive wound drainage, other discharge, or fecal incontinence. Transmission-based precautions include the following:

Contact	Use PPE, including gown and gloves, for all contacts with the patient or the patient's immediate environment.
Droplet	(Appropriate for influenza, streptococcus infection, pertussis, rhinovirus, and adenovirus and pathogens that remain viable and infectious for only short distances.) Use a mask while caring for the patient. Maintain the patient at a distance of >3 feet away from other patients (with a curtain separating them in an emergency department). Use a patient mask if transporting a patient.
Airborne	(Appropriate for measles, chickenpox, tuberculosis, and severe acute respiratory syndrome [SARS] because pathogens remain viable and infectious for long distances.) Use ≥N95 respirators (or masks) while caring for the patient. The patient should be placed in an airborne infection isolation room in an emergency department.

Hand hygiene and gloves

Hand hygiene should be done before eating, before and after direct contact with a patient's skin, after contact with any body fluids, after contact with inanimate objects in the patient's immediate vicinity, when moving hands from a dirty to a clean area, after removing gloves, and after using the restroom. Hand hygiene is carried out in the following two manners:

- Antiseptic soaps/detergents: For visible soiling, after exposure to diarrhea stool or a patient with diarrhea, before eating, and after using the restroom. Wet hands, apply product, rub hands together vigorously for 15 seconds, covering all surfaces, rinse hands with water, and use a disposable towel to dry.

- Alcohol-based hand sanitizers (the most effective way to kill bacteria): For all other situations. Apply product and rub hands together, including between the fingers, for about 20 seconds until skin surfaces are dry.

Gloves must be worn when touching any body fluids, nonintact skin, open wounds, or mucous membranes (eyes, mouth, nose); gloves should be changed when moving from a dirty area to a clean one or from one patient to another.

Personal protective equipment (PPE)

Personal protective equipment (PPE) should be readily available in the appropriate sizes for each EMS individual.

- Gowns: Should be worn for risk of splash or spray with body fluids (severe bleeding, childbirth) and should be fluid resistant.
- Eye protectors: Should be worn for risk of splash or spray with body fluids or contact with debris, such as at a worksite or in a collapsing building. Goggles should fit snugly and have antifog features. (Prescription eyeglasses do not take the place of goggles.)
- Face shields: Provide protection for face, eyes, nose, and mouth. These are preferred to goggles when there is risk of spray or splash of body fluids. They should wrap around and cover the forehead and extend to below the chin.
- Masks: Protect the nose and mouth from fluids and particles and should be fluid resistant, fit snugly, and have a flexible nosepiece.
- Respirators (such as N95, N99, and N100): Protect the nose, mouth, and airway passages exposed to hazardous or infectious aerosols, including microorganisms (tuberculosis [TB], measles).

Procedures for exposure/contamination

Any **exposure/contamination** should be reported at hand-off and to the appropriate infection control person, following protocols, and follow-up care should be sought if necessary. Decontamination procedures are as follows:

- Skin: Cleanse the area thoroughly with soap and water.
- Eyes: Flush with water for 20 minutes.
- Needlestick: Wash area with soap and water and report immediately.
- Clothing: Remove clothing as soon as possible, and wash visible soiling of skin with soap and water if a shower is not immediately available, but shower as soon as possible. Clothes should be washed separately in a washing machine at the workplace.
- Equipment/Vehicles: Clean thoroughly with disinfectant. Dispose of equipment if unable to adequately decontaminate it.

When reporting exposures/contamination, note the type of exposure, the date and time of exposure, circumstances, actions taken to decontaminate, and any other required information.

Dealing with stressful incidents

The EMR must often deal with **stressful incidents**, such as dangerous situations (storm conditions, gunshots, falling debris); critically ill patients; unpleasant sights, sounds, and odors; multipatient incidents; and angry/upset patients, family members, and bystanders. The EMR should not argue or become defensive but should remain calm and supportive, allowing the patient to express his or her feelings and trying to defuse the situation while administering medical care and cooperating with other first responders. If a patient has no pulse or respirations and does not have a valid do-not-resuscitate (DNR) order, the EMR should attempt resuscitation unless doing so puts the EMR at risk; the injuries are not compatible with life; or obvious signs of death are present, such as tissue decay, livor mortis, which is discoloration in the lowermost blood vessels from pooled blood shortly after death, or rigor mortis, which is stiffening of the joints that occurs within 2 to 6 hours of death (verified by checking two or more joints). After 24 to 48 hours of rigor mortis, the muscles become flaccid.

Warning signs of stress

Warning signs of stress often begin with difficulty sleeping and nightmares about work, loss of appetite, and lack of interest in usual activities, including work and intimacy. The individual may feel increasingly sad and depressed and may have difficulty concentrating, making decisions, and carrying out tasks. The individual may also begin to isolate from others and exhibit irritability with coworkers, family, and friends. Some individuals develop physical symptoms related to stress, such as stomach upset, headaches, nausea, and high blood pressure (BP), whereas others may experience panic attacks. Some individuals may try to self-medicate with alcohol or drugs. When experiencing the warning signs of stress, the individual should talk about the problems with someone trusted (such as a physician, coworker, supervisor, or family member), and he or she may need to seek assistance from a professional counselor. Lifestyle changes, such as decreasing the use of alcohol or drugs, exercising regularly, and practicing relaxation exercises, may help to relieve stress.

Kübler-Ross's five stages of grief

Grief is a normal response to the death or severe illness/abnormality of a patient. How a person deals with grief is very personal, and each will grieve differently. Elisabeth Kübler-Ross identified **five stages of grief**, which can apply to patients and to family members. A person may not go through each stage but usually goes through two of the five stages.

Stage	Patient/Family	Appropriate EMR response
1. Denial	Resistive to information, stunned, immobile, detached, unable to respond appropriately.	Be patient and supportive and repeat information as needed.
2. Anger	Lashing out, overt hostility, self-blame, blaming others.	Do not respond in anger or take statements personally; remain calm and supportive, but be alert to the risk of physical attack.
3. Bargaining	If–then thinking, demanding another opinion or expert, praying.	Avoid making any judgmental statements.
4. Depression	Tearful, crying, withdrawn, sad, isolated.	Encourage expression of feelings, remain supportive, and assure the individual that these feelings are normal.
5. Acceptance	Resolution.	Listen patiently and remain supportive.

Interpretation of signs and symbols

Sign/Symbol	Interpretation
	Flame: Includes flammable materials and gases and those that are self-heating or self-reactive.
	Corrosion: Includes substances that can cause skin burns, metal corrosion, and eye damage.
	Health hazard: Includes carcinogens, toxic substances, and respiratory irritants.
	Poison: Includes materials, gases, or substances that are extremely toxic and may result in death or severe illness.
	Irritant: Includes material, gases, or substances that are irritants to skin, eyes, and/or respiratory tract, are acutely toxic, or have a narcotic effect.
	Biohazard: Includes biological substances, such as body fluids, that pose a threat to humans. Appears on sharps containers that hold contaminated needles.

Basic principles of body mechanics

Basic principles of body mechanics include the following:

- Avoid reaching for prolonged periods of time, overhead, or more than 20 inches away.
- Avoid pulling—push, roll, or slide instead.
- Avoid lifting—push, roll, or slide instead.
- Lift with leg muscles, not with the back.
- Hold weight close to the body rather than at arm's length.
- Flex at the hips and knees, not the waist.
- Carry patients head first upstairs and feet first downstairs.
- Maintain a straight back and avoid twisting.
- Assess weight and recognize limitations in lifting/carrying.

- Get help when necessary, and communicate every step with your partner ("Lift on the count of three").
- Maintain a firm base of support with feet apart (shoulder width) to stabilize your stance.
- Maintain the line of gravity (the imaginary line between your center of gravity and the ground) within the base of support.
- Position yourself close to an object that is to be lifted or carried.
- Lift patients from stable ground.

Techniques for moving and lifting patients

Techniques for moving patients include the following:

- Direct ground lift: Use only for lightweight individuals with no suspected spinal injuries. Three rescuers line up on one side of the patient, and each kneels on the same knee. The EMR at the head places one arm under the patient's neck and shoulder and the other arm under the patient's lower back. The middle EMR places his or her arms above and below the patient's waist, and the EMR at the patient's feet places his or her arms under the knees and lower legs. On the count of three, they roll the patient onto their knees and toward their chests. On the count of three, they stand and move the patient.
- Power lift: Place feet shoulder width apart and pointing slightly outward; tighten the back and abdominal muscles. Squat down as though sitting. Place hands 10 inches apart with the palms upward (power grip) while grasping the stretcher and lift with the upper body becoming vertical before the hips rise.
- Extremity lift: Requires two EMRs. One EMR squats at the patient's head, and another is at one side by the patient's knees. The EMR at the head folds the patient's arms across the chest and grasps the patient by wrapping both arms around the torso under the patient's arms and grasping the patient's wrists. The second EMR slides his or her hands beneath the patient's knees and lower legs, and together they stand and lift the patient.
- Squat lift: Requires two EMRs. One EMR squats with the back straight and weak foot slightly forward at the head of patient, and the other EMR is in the same position at the patient's feet. Grasp the patient's upper body as for the extremity lift and grasp the feet. Both EMRs push up with the stronger foot and lift with the upper body becoming vertical before the hips rise.
- Logroll: Used to position carrying devices under a patient and for some transfers; it requires two EMRs positioned on the same side of the patient. Place the patient's arm on the side that he or she is being turned to above his or her head or over the chest. Place the patient's other arm across his or her chest. If on the ground, squat close to the patient. The EMR at the patient's head reaches across the patient and grasps his or her shoulders and trunk while the second EMR grasps his or her trunk and legs. On the count of three, they turn the patient in one smooth move.
- Draw-sheet transfer: Requires four EMRs with two positioned on one side of the patient and two positioned on the other side but on the opposite side of the bed or stretcher to which the patient will be transferred. The logroll technique is used to place a draw sheet under the patient. EMRs on both sides roll the edges of the draw sheet until the edges are close to the patient. On the count of three, they lift the patient slightly and move the patient across to the bed.

Emergency moves

Emergency moves may be needed if the patient and/or EMR is in immediate danger from fire, explosives, or other hazards; if the patient requires life-saving treatment, such as cardiopulmonary resuscitation (CPR); or if the patient is in water, such as a pond or lake. Emergency moves include the following:

- Blanket drag: Logroll the patient onto a blanket, wrap the patient in the blanket, grasp the blanket near the patient's head while in a squatting position with your back straight, and drag. If there are two rescuers, the other should be positioned at the patient's feet and should be pushing.
- Clothing drag: Squat down by the patient's head, securely grasp the clothing near the patient's neck or shoulders (avoid grasping by a T-shirt), and drag the patient.
- Arm drag: Squat down by the patient's head. Fold the patient's arms across his or her chest. Grasp the patient under the arms, wrapping your arms about the torso and grasping the patient's wrists to stabilize his or her arms. Drag the patient.

Urgent moves, such as with altered mental status, shock, or breathing difficulties, should also be done as quickly as possible.

Emergency moves can be carried out by one rescuer if no other assistance is available, as follows:

- Firefighter's drag: Tie the patient's wrists together with any available material. Straddle the patient and pull the patient's arms over your neck and then crawl forward, dragging him or her beneath you.
- Firefighter's carry: Grasp the patient's knees and pull them together and up. Stand on the patient's feet and reach out and grab one of the patient's arms with one hand. Pull the patient upright, and, as the patient elevates, place your other hand between the patient's legs. Place the patient's arm behind your neck and continue to pull the patient and lift until he or she is draped across your upper back with the arm hanging free. Then grasp the patient's arm that is hanging with the hand that is between the legs to secure the patient.

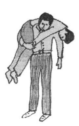

Restraints

Restraints should be avoided if possible, although if a combative patient poses a risk to him- or herself or EMS personnel, restraints may be necessary to safely assess, treat, and transport a patient, keeping in mind that the altered state of consciousness may result from drug or alcohol use; traumatic injury; or from a mental or physical disorder, such as schizophrenia, dementia, or hypoglycemia (insulin reaction). Protocols for use of restraints must be followed, and restraints should be applied under medical direction. If possible, the police should be present and there should be one EMS personnel for each limb, staying beyond the limb's range of motion until ready to secure the limb, with one EMR talking to the patient and explaining the procedure. The EMR should avoid unnecessary force, which may result in increased combativeness and injury to the patient or others. Patients should not be restrained in the prone (face-down) position.

Documentation must include the reason for restraining the patient, the time, and the method of restraint.

Common **types of physical restraints** include the following:

- Soft: Padded cuffs (often leather) that fasten about the wrists and ankles and are attached to a long board. These are the most commonly used restraints.
- Stretcher/Spinal board straps: These may be strapped across the chest (not too tight), abdomen, or legs to help restrict movement.
- Long board/Spinal board: Patient should be restrained to the long board and then placed on a wheeled stretcher and never tied to or fastened to the stretcher.
- Spit sock: A hood that fits over the patient's head to prevent him or her from biting or spitting.
- Cervical collar: This is used to protect the patient's cervical spine and to prevent him or her from biting.

The EMR should not place the patient in handcuffs or hard plastic ties. If these were placed on a patient by a law enforcement officer and must stay in place, such as with a criminal or an extremely violent patient, then a law enforcement officer must stay with the patient at all times.

Prevention of response-related injuries

Prevention of response-related injuries includes the following:

- Infectious diseases: Use PPE and understand the spread of infectious diseases—air (coughing), direct contact (blood, vomitus, other body fluids), needlesticks, contaminated food/equipment, and sexual transmission. Maintain current immunizations.
- Personal habits: Obtain adequate sleep, nutrition, and exercise. Avoid excessive alcohol and tobacco.
- Environmental hazards: Conduct a 360° assessment. Note traffic hazards, the vehicle's condition, fire, leaking fluids, downed power lines, hazardous materials (look for placards and warning symbols; avoid the area until it is cleared). Use PPE and respirators as indicated.
  - Violence: Defuse situations, make a safe response (with the assistance of law enforcement), and use restraints if necessary for dangerous or violent individuals.
- Collisions: Drive safely; avoid speeding and driving through stop signs and red lights when possible. Wear seat belts and/or safety harnesses.

Prehospital care report

The **prehospital care report** serves as a legal document to show that emergent care was provided and describes the condition of the patient on arrival at the scene, interventions, and changes in condition, and it is essential to ensure the continuity of care. The prehospital care report may also be used for educational purposes, such as through debriefing and case review. Additionally, the report is used administratively as the basis for billing as well as for the collection of data for research and evaluation of continuous quality improvement. Required elements of documentation include the time of events (receipt of call, arrival at incident, time of transport, arrival at destination), assessment findings (vital signs, injuries, bleeding, mental status), emergent care, changes in the patient's condition, response to the treatment provided, scene observations (specific place/area), hazards, and disposition of patient (care refusal, transportation, hand-off).

Documentation may be on paper or may be done electronically and may combine checkboxes and narrative reports.

EMS system communication

With the **EMR's arrival** at the scene of an incident, he or she should assess the situation and the need for added resources, such as additional EMS personnel or police, and contact the appropriate authorities to request assistance. When additional EMS personnel arrive or contact is made with medical control or the receiving facility, the EMR should self-identify and provide a verbal report of the patient's current condition, including demographic information such as age and gender. The EMR should report the patient's chief complaint and provide any history that is pertinent as well as the condition of the patient on arrival and any history of major illnesses. The EMR should also report the results of the patient assessment, including the vital signs and any physical/psychological findings, as well as any treatment provided and the patient's response to the treatment. The EMR should communicate with law enforcement officers and other responders, such as firefighters, especially regarding safety concerns.

Effective communication and interviewing techniques

Effective communication begins with a self-introduction and an introduction of other team members to the patient and family and respecting the patient's privacy by shielding the patient from passersby if possible and avoiding loudly repeating any patient information. If possible, the EMR should adjust lighting and limit outside distractions such as noise. When interviewing the patient, the EMR should ask open-ended questions (such as "Can you describe your pain?") and avoid questions that can be answered with "yes" or "no." The EMR should ask direct questions, such as "When did the pain start?" Questions should be asked one at a time while allowing the patient/family time to respond. It's especially important to observe the patient's body language (posture, eye contact, gestures, tone of voice) to determine if it matches his or her words and to avoid medical/professional jargon. The EMR should avoid giving false reassurances or advice and should avoid leading/biased questions, being too talkative, interrupting the patient, and asking "why" questions, such as "Why did you take an overdose of medication?"

Cultural competence

There are a number of issues related to cultural competence in communicating with others.

- **Eye contact:** Many cultures use eye contact differently than what is common in the United States. Some patients or families, such as Asians, Native Americans, and Arabs, may avoid direct eye contact, considering it rude, or they may look away to signal disapproval or may look down to signal respect. Careful observation of the way family members use eye contact can help to determine what will be most comfortable for the patient/family.
- **Distance**: Some cultures stand close to others (<4 feet) when speaking (Middle Easterners, Hispanics), and others stand at a greater distance (>4 feet) (Northern Europeans, many Americans). There is a considerable difference relating to concepts of personal space among cultures. Allowing the family to approach or observing whether they tend to move closer, lean forward, or move back can help to determine a comfortable distance for communication.
- **Time**: Americans tend to be time oriented, and they expect people to be on time, but time is viewed more flexibly in many other cultures.

Therapeutic communication

Therapeutic communication begins with respect for the individual/family and the assumption that all communication, verbal and nonverbal, has meaning. Listening must be done empathetically. Techniques that facilitate communication include the following:

Introduction	Make a personal introduction and use the individual's name: "Mrs. Brown, I am Toby Williams, your EMR."
Encouragement	Use an open-ended opening question: "Is there anything you'd like to discuss?" Acknowledge comments: Say "yes" and "I understand." Allow silence and observe nonverbal behavior rather than trying to force a conversation. Ask for clarification if the patient's statements are unclear. Reflect the patient's statements back (use sparingly): Individual: "I hate this hospital." EMR: "You hate this hospital?"
Empathy	Make observations: "You are shaking," and "You seem worried." Recognize feelings: Individual: "I want to get well." EMR: "It must be hard for you to deal with this illness." Provide information as honestly and completely as possible about the patient's condition, treatment, and procedures and respond to the individual's questions and concerns.
Exploration	Verbally express implied messages: Individual: "This treatment is too much trouble." EMR: "Do you think the treatment isn't helping you?" Explore a topic, but allow the individual to terminate the discussion without further probing: "I'd like to hear how you feel about that."
Orientation	Indicate reality: Individual: "Someone is screaming." EMR: "That sound was a police siren." Comment on distortions without directly agreeing or disagreeing: Individual: "That policeman promised I could go to St. John's Hospital." EMR: "Really? That's surprising because this ambulance is based at County Hospital."
Collaboration	Work together to achieve better results: "Maybe if we talk about this, we can figure out a way to make the treatment easier for you."
Validation	Seek validation: "Do you feel better now?" or "Did the medication help you breathe better?"

Interviewing techniques

If possible, the patient should be interviewed alone or should be asked if he/she wants family members present. Verbal and nonverbal responses should be observed during **an interview**. Information should include not only patient's facts but also patient's attitude and concerns. The

EMR should ask one question at a time in language that the patient understands and avoid providing false reassurances and advice or interrupting. Strategies include the following:

- Ask open-ended informational questions (as opposed to yes/no) with "who," "what," "where," "when," and "how," but avoid questions with "why" if possible.
- Instead of "Why do you continue to use heroin?" ask, "Have you tried to quit drug use?"
- Ask brief, clarifying questions: "How long have you had weakness in your left side?"
- Provide a list of options: "Is your headache throbbing, stabbing, or dull?"
- Rephrase/reflect to encourage clarification.
  - o Patient: "My husband had the same type of fall and died a month later."
  - o EMR: "You're afraid you might die from this fall."

Conditions for consent

The **conditions for consent** for care and decision-making capacity include the following:

- 18 years or older: Those who are younger may have the right to give consent for all or some medical treatment in some states. Laws vary. For example, the age of consent for medical treatment in Alabama is 14.
- Mentally competent to make decisions: May be impaired by mental disability, injury, illness, or substance abuse (intoxication).
- Court-emancipated minor.
- Military service.
- Marriage.

Consent may be expressed if the patient is able to give informed consent, or it may be implied, such as when care is provided in an emergent situation in which the patient is unable to give consent. Parents or caregivers give consent for minors younger than the age of 18 unless they have been emancipated. If parents or caregivers are unavailable to give consent, life-saving emergent care, general medical assessment, and medical care to prevent further injury or harm can be provided without consent.

Health Insurance Portability and Accountability Act of 1996 (HIPAA)

Sensitive information is classified under the **Health Insurance Portability and Accountability Act of 1996** (HIPAA) as protected health information (PHI), and it includes the following:

- Any information about an individual's past, present, or future health or condition (mental or physical).
- Provision of health care.
- Any identifying information related to payment for healthcare services.
- Identifying information: Name, address, Social Security number, birth date, and any document or material that contains the identifying information.

Personal information can be shared with a spouse, legal guardians, those with durable power of attorney for the patient, and those involved in the care of the patient, such as physicians, without a specific release.

HIPAA mandates the following privacy and security rules to ensure that health information and individual privacy are protected:

- <u>Privacy rule:</u> Protected information includes any information included in the medical record (electronic or paper), conversations between the doctor and other healthcare providers, billing information, and any other form of health information.
- <u>Security rule:</u> Any electronic health information must be secure and protected against threats, hazards, or nonpermitted disclosure.

Informed consent

Patients or their families must provide **informed consent** for all treatment they receive. This includes a thorough explanation of all procedures and treatment and associated risks. Patients/families should be apprised of all options and allowed input on the type of treatments. Patients/families should be apprised of all reasonable risks and any complications that might be life threatening or increase morbidity. The American Medical Association has established guidelines for informed consent as follows:

- Explanation of diagnosis.
- Nature of and reason for treatment or procedure.
- Risks and benefits.
- Alternative options (regardless of cost or insurance coverage).
- Risks and benefits of alternative options.
- Risks and benefits of not having a treatment or procedure.
- Providing informed consent is a requirement of all states.

The requirement for informed consent may be waived in life-threatening situations and if the EMR cannot obtain informed consent because the patient cannot communicate and legal consent cannot be obtained.

Advance directives, durable power of attorney, and do-not-resuscitate (DNR) order

In accordance with federal and state laws, individuals have the right to self-determination in health care, including decisions about end-of-life care through **advance directives** such as living wills and the right to assign a surrogate person to make decisions through a **durable power of attorney**. Patients should routinely be questioned about an advanced directive because they may present at a healthcare organization without the document. Patients who have indicated they desire a **do-not-resuscitate (DNR) order** should not receive resuscitative treatments for terminal illness or conditions in which meaningful recovery cannot occur. Patients and families of those with terminal illnesses should be questioned as to whether the patients are hospice patients. For those with DNR requests or those withdrawing life support, healthcare providers should provide the patient palliative rather than curative measures, such as pain control and/or oxygen, and emotional support to the patient and family. Religious traditions and beliefs about death should be treated with respect.

Patient Self-Determination Act

According to the **Patient Self-Determination Act** (1990), competent patients have the right to **refusal of care**, and parents have the right to make this decision for minor children. If a patient refuses care, then the EMR should try to persuade the patient to go to the hospital by giving the reasons and possible consequences of refusal. The patient should be asked to sign the refusal form and a family member, police officer, or bystander should sign as a witness to the patient's signing or witness the refusal to sign. The EMR should complete documentation of any assessment carried out and any refusal of the patient to assessment. The EMR should carefully document the conversation between the EMR and patient regarding refusal of care and consequences and should document the proposed care as well as the information the EMR gave the patient about alternate care (such as a visit to the personal physician) and the willingness to return if the patient has a change of mind.

Civil and criminal offenses related to patient care

The four necessary elements of **negligence** (failure to follow the standards of care) are as follows:

1. Duty of care: The defendant (healthcare provider) had a duty to provide adequate care and/or protect the plaintiff's (patient's) safety.
2. Breach of duty: The defendant failed to carry out the duty to care, resulting in danger, injury, or harm to the plaintiff.
3. Damages: The plaintiff experienced illness or injury as a result of the breach of duty.
4. Causation: The plaintiff's illness or injury is directly caused by the defendant's negligent breach of duty.

Abandonment occurs if the EMR withdraws from providing care contrary to patient's desire or knowledge and fails to arrange for appropriate care by others, resulting in harm to the patient. **Assault** occurs if an EMR threatens a patient in such a way that the patient becomes fearful of harm, whereas **battery** occurs when the EMR intentionally injures a patient, such as by hitting or shoving the person. Assault and battery often occur together.

Negligence

Negligence indicates that *proper care* has not been provided, based on established standards. *Reasonable care* uses a rationale for decision making in relation to providing care. State regulations regarding negligence may vary, but all have some statutes of limitation, governmental immunity, and Good Samaritan laws that may provide a defense. Types of negligence include the following:

- Negligent conduct: Failure to provide reasonable care or to protect/assist another, based on standards and expertise.
- Gross negligence: Willfully providing inadequate care while disregarding the safety and security of another.
- Contributory negligence: Injured party contributes to his/her own harm.
- Comparative negligence: The percentage amount of negligence attributed to each individual involved.

If the charge of negligence is supported, the patient may collect physical (lost earnings due to injury), psychological (pain and suffering), and punitive damages.

Statutory responsibilities and mandatory reporting

The EMR must practice within the **scope of responsibility**, which is outlined by each state's medical practice act. The EMR must be certified/licensed according to state requirements and meet appropriate educational standards regarding preparation and continuing education. The EMR has a duty to the patients, the medical director, and the public and functions under government and medical oversight.

Although laws about **mandatory reporting** vary from state to state, healthcare providers, including EMS personnel, are considered mandatory reporters in all states and must report suspected cases of child and elder abuse and neglect. The EMR must follow state guidelines for reporting because simply notifying the receiving facility of suspected abuse or neglect is not adequate. The EMR should be familiar with the signs of abuse and neglect (certain types of fractures; unexplained or multiple bruises; suspicious bruise patterns; burns; hair loss; and inadequate food, clothing, and shelter).

Evidence preservation

When an incident may involve **court cases**, such as with gunshot wounds, knife wounds, and rape, the EMR should take steps to preserve evidence, although providing emergent medical care takes priority. The EMR should try to avoid disturbing items at the scene of the incident and should assess the environment and document any unusual findings, remembering that the environment and the patient are both considered to be part of the crime scene. The EMR should collaborate with law enforcement officers at the scene. If the patient has had a gunshot wound or knife wound, the EMR should not cut through the holes in the clothing but should cut along seams or away from the injuries. Any clothing or belongings removed during treatment should be secured separately in a paper bag (or plastic if paper is not available) and delivered with the patient to the receiving facility or to the law enforcement officers. When the patient is describing the event, the EMR should document quotations rather than summarizing.

Ethical principles and moral obligations

Ethics is a branch of philosophy that studies morality—concepts of right and wrong. Applied ethics is the use of ethical principles, such as autonomy (right to self-determination), beneficence (acting to benefit another), nonmaleficence (doing no harm), verity (being truthful), and justice (equally distributing resources/care). Ethical conflicts may occur because of differences in cultural and ethical values, but they may also result from decisions that must be made regarding care, such as whether to provide CPR in a wilderness situation when the treatment is likely futile, situations involving triage in which some patients are given priority over others, situations that involve professional misconduct (such as EMS personnel being abusive toward patients), and incidents of patient dumping because the patient has inadequate insurance or ability to pay. EMS personnel have a moral obligation to make decisions about care in good faith and in the patient's best interest.

Decision-making models

Decision-making models	
Do no harm	This model is based on nonmaleficence, the requirement that a treatment provided do no harm; however, by their nature, some treatments can and often do harm patients, so the underlying intent and goal of treatment must be considered when making decisions. For example, CPR may be carried out to save a patient's life and may be done with correct technique but still may result in rib fractures.
In good faith	The motive for a decision should be honest and fair, and decisions should be made with a sincere intention to do good even though the outcome may be negative. For example, EMS personnel may provide a treatment for a patient in good faith although the treatment proves to be ineffective for that particular patient.

| Patient's best interest | Making a decision in the patient's best interest includes considering the patient's or parents' (in the case of children) wishes, the best clinical judgment, the best choice of various options, the chances for improvement/decline, and religious/cultural preferences. |

Anatomy and Physiology

Anatomic terms

Commonly used **anatomic terms** include the following:

- Anterior: Situated toward the front.
- Posterior: Situated toward the back.
- Superior: Situated above.
- Inferior: Situated below.
- Midline: In the middle.
- Medial: Situated toward the midline.
- Lateral: Situated toward the side, away from the midline.
- Distal: Farthest from the point of reference.
- Proximal: Closest to the point of reference.

When describing an area of the patient's body, the description should be patient oriented, using phrases such as "patient's left" and "patient's right" to ensure accurate interpretation.

Medical Terminology

Common medical prefixes

Term	Meaning	Examples
Cardio-	Heart	Cardiovascular (heart and vessels), cardiology (study of the heart)
Neuro-	Nerves	Neurology (study of the nerves), neuron (nerve cell)
Hyper-	Enlarged, excessive, high	Hypertrophy (enlarged tissue), hyperemesis (excessive vomiting), hyperactive (overactive), hypertension (high BP)
Hypo-	Under, beneath, low	Hypoglycemia (low blood sugar), hypotension (low BP), hypoxia (low oxygen)
Naso-	Nose	Nasopharyngeal (nose and throat), nasal (referring to the nose)
Oro-	Mouth	Oropharyngeal (mouth and throat), oral (referring to the mouth)
Arterio-	Artery	Arteriovenous (artery and vein), arterial (referring to arteries)
Hemo- **Hemato**	Blood	Hemolysis (breakdown of blood), hemoglobin (blood component), hematology (study of blood)
Therm-	Temperature	Thermoregulation (temperature regulation), thermometer (temperature measurement)
Vaso-	Vessels	Vasoconstriction (narrowing of vessels), vasodilation (widening of vessels)
Tachy-	Rapid	Tachycardia (rapid heart rate), tachypnea (rapid respirations)
Brady-	Slow	Bradycardia (slow heart rate), bradypnea (slow respirations)

Pathophysiology

Respiratory compromise

Respiratory compromise may relate to problems with the following:

- Airway: The airway is blocked because of a foreign body, the tongue (especially in unconscious patients and young children), blood or secretions, edema (swelling), or trauma (blunt or penetrating).
- Respirations: The patient is unable to adequately breathe in enough oxygen because of inadequate oxygen in environment, poison gases (such as carbon monoxide), lung infection (pneumonia), illness that narrows breathing passages (chronic obstructive pulmonary disease [COPD], bronchitis), excess fluid in the lungs (pulmonary edema), excess fluid between the lung tissue and the blood vessels (leaving inadequate blood volume), and impaired circulation.
- Ventilation: Rate or depth of breathing is inadequate for air exchange; volume of air breathed in is too small; air exchange is impaired by altered consciousness, unconsciousness, chest injury, overdose of medication (such as narcotics), poisoning, and disease (such as amyotrophic lateral sclerosis [ALS], sometimes called Lou Gehrig's disease).

Shock

Shock, which is impaired blood flow to the body tissues (cells and organs) may relate to problems with the following:

- Heart: If the heart rate is too slow or too rapid and contractions are ineffectual, insufficient blood is pumped to the lungs for oxygenation and to the cells and body organs. Heart problems may relate to heart disease (such as heart failure), poisoning, and artificial ventilation that is excessive or ineffective.
- Blood vessels: Blood vessels may be unable to constrict, resulting in vasodilation and lowering of BP. This most often occurs because of cervical (neck) spinal cord injuries, severe infection, or anaphylactic reaction.
- Blood: The volume of circulating blood or blood components may be inadequate to nurture the body cells and organs because of excessive bleeding or vomiting, diarrhea, or burns, which may result in dehydration.

Life Span Development

Normal vital signs from neonate to older adulthood

Age	Heart rate	Respirations	BP (mm Hg)
Neonate (newborn)	100–220 (average 140–160) begins to slow after 3 months	40–60 for a few minutes, then 30–40	Systolic 70–90
Toddler (12–36 mos.)	80–130	20–30	Systolic 70–100
Preschool (3 to 5)	80–120	20–30	Systolic 80–110
School age (6–12)	70–110	20–30	80–120/60–80
Adolescence (13–18)	55–100	12–20	110–131/64–84
Early adulthood (19–40)	60–100 (average 80)	12–20	100–119/60–79 to 140/90 (high BP)
Middle adulthood (41–60)	60–100 (average 80)	12–20	100–119/60–79 to 140/90 (high BP)
Late adulthood (61+)	60–100 (average 70)	12–20	100–119/60–79 to 140/90 (high BP)

Growth and development of pediatric patients

Age	Characteristics
0–2 mos.	Sleeps up to 16 hours a day but should rouse easily. Cries for a reason, and persistent crying may indicate illness. Limited head control. Gazes at faces.
2–6 mos.	Smiles voluntarily and makes eye contact, uses both hands, begins to hold head up, rolls over, and sleeps through the night.
6–12 mos.	Sits, crawls, has pincer grasp, mouths objects (increasing risk of poisoning and aspiration), babbles, and speaks first words by 12 months. Exhibits separation anxiety from parents.
12–18 mos.	Begins to walk; imitates others; knows body parts and 4–6 words; lacks molars for grinding food, increasing the risk of aspiration; and has increased mobility.
18–24 mos.	Begins to run and climb, knows 100 words (24 months), clings to parents, attaches to special objects, labels objects, and begins to understand cause and effect.
2–5 years	Walks, runs, throws, catches, is toilet trained, has magical thinking and irrational fears, learns acceptable behavior, has temper tantrums, and develops modesty.
6–12 years	Loses baby teeth; thinks logically; becomes self-conscious; understands the finality of death; attaches importance to school, popularity, and peers.
12–20 years	Puberty begins, reasons (imperfectly), is self-conscious, seeks independence and peer approval, and takes risks.

Public Health

Levels of disease prevention

Levels of disease prevention include the following:

- Primary: The goal is to prevent the initial occurrence of a health problem, such as a disease or injury, through such activities as immunizations, smoking cessation, fluoride supplementation of water, promotion of seat belt and helmet use, and use of child car seat restraints. Interventions are often aimed at the general public or large groups of people.
- Secondary: The goal is to identify diseases or conditions quickly and provide prompt intervention to provide treatment and prevent further disability through such activities as BP screenings, breast and testicular self-examinations, hearing and vision screenings, mammography, and pregnancy testing.
- Tertiary: The goal is to assist those who already have disease or disability to prevent further progression of the disease and to allow people to achieve the maximum quality of life through such activities as support groups, counseling, diet and exercise, stress management, and supportive services.

Safety equipment

Safety equipment may include a wide variety of devices, including smoke alarms and carbon monoxide alarms. Some safety equipment protects people from falls, especially older adults. These may include safety rails, grab bars, canes, and walkers. EMS personnel are often involved in public education regarding the following:

- Car seats: Should be properly secured in the back seat of a motor vehicle. They should be rear facing for infants and toddlers up to 2 years of age (or the maximum recommended height and weight) and forward facing with a harness for toddlers and preschoolers. School-aged children should use booster seats with a belt and harness until they are at least 4 feet 9 inches tall. Children younger than age 13 should not ride in a front seat.
- Seat belts: All people in a motor vehicle should be secured with seat belts and shoulder harnesses.
- Helmets: Should fit properly and snugly, cover the top of the forehead, and have a securing chin strap. They should be worn when riding a bicycle or motorcycle and engaging in sports activities such as rollerblading but not on playground equipment or when climbing trees.

Airway Management, Respirations and Artificial Ventilation

Life support chain

Critical to the **life support chain** are oxygenation and perfusion. Oxygenation involves gas exchange of carbon dioxide for oxygen at the alveolar/capillary level and the cell/capillary level. Perfusion involves the transport of blood, which oxygen, glucose, and other nutrients as well as waste products throughout the body. Oxygen and glucose are essential for cell functioning. Glucose is produced by the digestion of carbohydrates (starches); it is the primary energy source for the body; and its use is controlled by insulin, which is produced by the pancreas. Excess glucose is stored in the liver as glycogen for later use or is converted to fat. These fundamental elements are affected by the composition of ambient air (usually 21% oxygen), airway patency, ventilation, regulation of respiration, blood volume and transport, heart action, and blood vessel size and resistance.

Respiratory (airway) system

Air enters the **respiratory system** through the nose and mouth, where it is warmed and moistened, and it passes through the pharynx (the back of the throat) and the larynx (voice box) into the trachea (windpipe). The epiglottis is a cartilage flap that closes over the larynx when swallowing so food enters the esophagus (the tube leading to the stomach). The trachea branches into right and left bronchi (large tubes) that carry the air into the lungs. Each bronchus branches into smaller bronchioles and millions of alveoli (small air sacs), which are covered with webs of tiny capillaries that deliver carbon dioxide and pick up oxygen (external respiration). Muscles of respiration are the diaphragm and the intercostal muscles (between the ribs), but accessory muscles in the neck and collarbone area may help during respiratory distress. The heart circulates unoxygenated blood to the lungs. After oxygenation, the blood returns to the heart and into the general circulation and body cells where gas exchange occurs again (internal respiration). Cells intake oxygen and nutrients and release carbon dioxide and waste products (cellular respiration).

Differences in the respiratory system associated with pediatric patients and older adults:

- **Pediatrics:** Infants are obligate nasal breathers for their first two to four months of life, and they usually only breathe through the nose, although they can generally breathe through the mouth if necessary. However, if nasal passages are blocked, they may quickly develop respiratory distress. Chest wall compliance is greater in infants and small children, so they must work harder than an adult to move the same amount of air. Additionally, proportionally the airway is smaller, the tongue is larger, and the cartilage is softer, increasing the risk of obstruction.
- **Older adults:** Breathing capacity tends to decline after age 40 because the number of alveoli decreases and the size of alveoli increases, resulting in less surface for and less efficient gas exchange. Lung elasticity also decreases, resulting in decreased vital capacity. The chest muscles tend to weaken and stiffen with age, and older adults have a lowered ability to cough and clear the airways.

Airway assessment and manual measures to clear the airway

Indications of an adequate airway include a normal voice and speaking ability and audible and visible air exchange. Indications of **inadequate airway** include unusual breathing sounds (wheezing, stridor), hoarse voice/inability to speak, and/or no audible or visible air exchange. Airway obstruction may result from the tongue falling back, food, a foreign body, vomit, blood, teeth, and edema (swelling). Maneuvers include the following:

- Head tilt/chin lift: Hyperextend the neck by tilting the head back with one hand on the patient's forehead to straighten the airway and lift the tongue. Then lift the chin and pull forward with the fingers of the other hand under the chin and with the thumb on top. The chin lift pulls the mandible (jaw) forward. This prevents the tongue from blocking the pharynx. Contraindications to the head tilt/chin lift include suspected cervical spine and neck injuries.
- Jaw thrust: This technique is used with a suspected spinal cord or neck injury in which extending the neck must be avoided. From behind, place your fingers behind the angles of the patient's lower jaw and place your thumbs on the patient's chin; move the jaw upward until it is extended while using the thumbs to slightly open the patient's mouth. Contraindications include severe facial injuries.
- Modified chin lift/jaw thrust: This technique is used with a suspected spinal cord/neck injury with an unstable cervical spine. From the head of the patient, place your thumbs on his or her cheekbones and place your fingers under the patient's mandible, and then pull the mandible upward with the fingers while applying pressure with the thumbs. If using a mask for ventilation, place the mask in position and secure it with your thumbs while your fingers thrust the patient's jaw forward.

Oropharyngeal (OPA) airway

The **oropharyngeal airway** (OPA), a blind-insertion airway device, may be inserted to provide better ventilation, but the OPA requires the head tilt/chin lift or modified jaw thrust as well because the device alone does not ensure a patent airway. The OPA is indicated for unconscious patients, patients with no gag reflex, and patients who are apneic (not breathing) and require ventilatory aid. The OPA is often inserted if a patient stops breathing, such as with a cardiac arrest. The OPA is contraindicated in conscious patients and those with a gag reflex. To insert the OPA, perform the following steps:

- Estimate the length of the OPA by measuring the patient from the angle of the jaw or the tip of the earlobe to the corner of the mouth.
- Select the correct size.
- Open the patient's mouth using the cross-finger technique. Suction any secretions.
- Tilt the head back (if possible). Insert the device with the tip of the OPA pointing upward.
- Rotate the OPA into position.
- Ensure that the phalanges of the mouthpiece are securely against the patient's mouth..
- Check to make sure that the OPA is patent (open).

Suctioning

Suctioning devices may be vehicle mounted or portable and should be checked to ensure that the tubing is intact and the canister has an airtight seal. Patients at risk for aspiration include those with an altered level of consciousness, those having difficulty swallowing or breathing, trauma patients, obese patients, and those with recurrent vomiting. Oral suctioning is used to remove secretions, vomitus, and blood. Suctioning may be done with a rigid-tip catheter (Yankauer) or a soft-tip catheter.

Techniques include the following:

- Don a mask and gloves.
- Measure the patient from the tip of the ear to the corner of the mouth to determine how far to insert the catheter.
- Turn on the suction.
- Use the cross-finger technique to open the mouth.
- Insert the tube and apply suction. The rigid catheter has a finger control to start and stop suction.
- Move the catheter around the gum line and over the tongue to the back of the mouth, but avoid stimulating the gag reflex.
- Suction for no longer than 15 seconds at a time.
- Note: Clear a small infant's airway by suctioning the nose with a bulb syringe.

Portable oxygen cylinders

Two commonly used sizes of **portable oxygen cylinders** are D tanks (M15; 350 liters) and E tanks (M24; 625 liters). The EMR should use protective equipment (goggles, gloves). The cylinder should be placed upright. A label over the holes on the top of the cylinder indicates that the cylinder is full. Remove the label, leaving the washers in place unless the washers are built into the regulator. Face the opening of the tank away and use the key to crack the cylinder by letting out a small amount of oxygen. Apply the regulator and slide it into place. Tighten and then open the cylinder to check for pressure (there should be at least 200 psi). Close the cylinder, attach the oxygen tubing to the regulator, set the oxygen flow to the correct amount of liters, and then open the cylinder and administer oxygen to the patient. When discontinuing use of the cylinder, turn off the cylinder, remove the oxygen tubing, turn the oxygen flow setting up to bleed air from the regulator, and remove the regulator.

Physiology of respiration

The **physiology of respiration** includes the following:

- Ventilation: Movement of air in and out of the lungs during inhalation and exhalation. The normal tidal volume (air exchange when breathing normally) for an adult is about 500 mL, but it is lower for infants and children (5–7 mL/kg for neonates, 6–8 mL/kg for children). Breathing may be impaired by disease (muscular dystrophy), drugs, trauma, bronchoconstriction, allergic reactions, foreign body obstructions, and infection.
- Oxygenation: The process by which oxygen molecules bind to hemoglobin in the blood.. The blood saturation level reflects the amount of oxygen that is dissolved in the blood and available to body tissues, and it should be ≥95%.
- Respiration: The process by which the lungs exchange carbon dioxide for oxygen in the alveoli and provide this oxygenated blood to body tissues. Respiration may be external (inspiration, expiration), internal (exchange of gas) or cellular (cells perform tasks that require oxygen and glucose [sugar] and produce carbon dioxide as a waste product). Respiration may be impaired by a lack of air, toxins/poisons, and ineffective circulation (shock, cardiac arrest).

Assessment of respirations and supplemental oxygen administration

When **assessing respirations**, the EMR should note the patient's gag reflex and rate of respirations (whether it is normal for the patient's age or it is too fast, too slow, or absent). The EMR should also evaluate the rise and fall of the chest and any abnormal movements (such as sternal retraction, nasal [nose] flaring) noisy breathing (gurgling, wheezing), the use of accessory muscles, or the tripod position (sitting, leaning forward, and supporting the body with the hands). If breathing is abnormal or the pulse oximetry is less than 95%, the EMR should take precautions against bloodstream infection (BSI) and administer **supplemental oxygen** with a nonrebreather mask with the oxygen set at 12–15 L. The reservoir bag of the mask must be completely filled before applying the mask to the patient, securing it with an elastic band about the head. If the patient cannot tolerate the nonrebreather mask, then a nasal cannula may be used with the oxygen flow set at 4–6 L, the prongs inserted into the nostrils, and tubing secured by looping over the ears and tightening under the chin.

Assessment of oxygenation

Assessment of oxygenation includes the following:

- Evaluate respirations: Note the following signs of respiratory distress—rapid breathing, slow breathing, use of accessory muscles, nasal flaring, and sternal retraction—because they may indicate inadequate oxygenation.
- Assess mental status: Confusion may be associated with hypo-oxygenation (low oxygen), but it's important to determine a baseline mental status if possible because the patient may have dementia or may be confused because of medications.
- Assess skin: Note cyanosis (blue tinge) especially around the mouth, fingertips, and oral mucous membranes because this indicates a lack of oxygen. Another sign is pallor. Mottling of the skin, purplish or reddish discoloration especially on knees and feet, indicates hypo-oxygenation and is a common indication that death is near.
- DoMonitor pulse oximetry: It should be 95%–100%. If a patient has mild respiratory disease, the pulse oximetry level may be as low as 90% and still be within the normal range for the patient. Readings less than 90%–92% indicate hypoxemia (low oxygen in the blood).

Assessment of ventilation

Ventilation is adequate if the respiratory rate, depth of respiration, and effort of breathing are normal. Signs of inadequate ventilation include the following:

- Increased effort of breathing: Nasal flaring, sternal retraction (infants), use of abdominal or intercostal (between ribs) muscles, sweating, sitting in the tripod position (upright, leaning forward, hands on knees).
- Abnormal breath sounds: Wheezes, rales (crackles), and/or rhonchi (snoring/whistling sounds).
- Abnormal depth of breathing: Hypoventilation (too shallow) or hyperventilation (too deep).
- Abnormal rate of breathing: Tachypnea (too fast) or bradypnea (too slow).
- Abnormal chest wall movement: Splinting, asymmetric, paradoxical (chest wall/diaphragm move in during inhalation and out during exhalation—opposite of normal).
- Irregular breathing pattern: May include periods of apnea (no breathing).

Patients with inadequate ventilation or apnea in which there is no breathing or only occasional gasping require ventilation assistance, such as with a pocket mask or bag-valve mask (BVM).

Pocket-mask ventilation

Pocket-mask ventilation is used when administering cardiopulmonary resuscitation (CPR) to a patient who is in cardiac arrest and apneic (not breathing). If two EMS personnel are available, one should be positioned at the patient's head to administer pocket-mask ventilation while the other does compressions. If there is only one EMS personnel, then that person should be positioned at the patient's side.

Administration is as follows:

- Remove the mask from the container and push the flattened mask to open.
- Wipe the face clean with an alcohol swab if necessary to remove secretions, vomitus.
- Do a chin tilt or jaw thrust and place the mask over the nose and mouth, holding it in place with both hands to seal it tightly.
- Take a deep breath and blow in through the one-way valve, watching the chest rise to ensure that ventilation has occurred.
- Continue to ventilate the patient at a rate of 30 compressions to 2 ventilations for CPR.
- Attach supplemental oxygen if available to improve oxygenation.
- Upon patient recovery or completion of CPR, remove the mask, discard the valve, and disinfect the mask.

Bag-valve mask (BVM) ventilation

Bag-valve mask (BVM) ventilation equipment used for positive-pressure ventilation (PPV) includes a mask, a ventilator bag, an oxygen reservoir bag, and an attachment for oxygen delivery. The correct mask size is important: The mask should not cover the chin. BVM is contraindicated if the airway is not patent, but it is used for abnormal breathing and for respiratory distress/failure. BVM requires two EMS personnel—one to control the mask and the other to control the bag. Steps are as follows:

- Position behind patient's head and place the mask over the patient's nose and mouth and make a tight seal by holding it in place with your thumbs and index fingers while your other fingers slide under the patient's jaw to lift the chin.
- Squeeze the bag with inhalations initially for 5 to 10 breaths and then adjust the rate to at least 12 breaths per minute, slowly adjusting the rate and tidal volume delivered.

Assessment of lung compliance (the ability to expand and contract) includes observation of chest movement, rate of respirations, and feel of BVM. Difficult ventilation suggests impaired compliance. Note: The BVM can be used with or without oxygen.

Sellick's maneuver (cricoid pressure)

Sellick's maneuver (cricoid pressure) may be used with PPV to prevent air from flowing down the esophagus and into the stomach rather than down the trachea and into the lungs because stomach distension increases the risk of vomiting. This maneuver may also be used with intubation to prevent regurgitation of stomach contents and aspiration. Sellick's maneuver may be used on unconscious patients receiving a mask or BVM. The procedure consists of applying pressure downward to the cricoid cartilage of the neck (which is at the bottom of the larynx and blocks the upper esophagus) with the thumb and index finger. Pressure is usually applied at 30 to 40 newtons but no greater than 40 newtons because too great of force may block the airway. The maneuver may also cause nausea and vomiting and, with severe pressure, may result in rupture of the esophagus. Vomiting is a contraindication.

Positioning and use of the recovery position

The **recovery position** is used for patients who are unconscious but breathing (such as those with a drug overdose or after a seizure) and have no life-threatening injuries. This position helps to maintain a patent airway and reduces the risk of aspiration from vomitus.

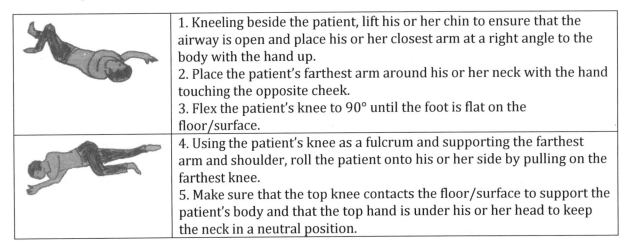

	1. Kneeling beside the patient, lift his or her chin to ensure that the airway is open and place his or her closest arm at a right angle to the body with the hand up. 2. Place the patient's farthest arm around his or her neck with the hand touching the opposite cheek. 3. Flex the patient's knee to 90° until the foot is flat on the floor/surface.
	4. Using the patient's knee as a fulcrum and supporting the farthest arm and shoulder, roll the patient onto his or her side by pulling on the farthest knee. 5. Make sure that the top knee contacts the floor/surface to support the patient's body and that the top hand is under his or her head to keep the neck in a neutral position.

Normal negative-pressure breathing and positive-pressure breathing

Negative-pressure breathing (normal)	Positive-pressure breathing
The movement downward of the diaphragm (triggered by the phrenic nerves) creates a negative pressure in the lungs, drawing air into them. Blood flows from the lungs to the heart and back and to the body at a steady rate in normal breathing. The epiglottis closes the esophagus during inhalation, preventing air from entering the stomach.	Ventilation forces air into the lungs, and this can result in dysfunction of the diaphragm because it is responding to a change in pressure rather than stimulation by the phrenic nerve. Blood flow from the lungs is reduced, resulting in decreased cardiac (heart) output. The epiglottis may stay open during ventilation, allowing air into the stomach and increasing the risk of vomiting.

Assessment

Primary assessment on arrival at a scene

After surveying the environment for safety issues, the EMR should quickly conduct a **primary assessment** to identify conditions that are life threatening, as follows:

- Level of consciousness: Alert, responsive to verbal stimuli, responsive to painful stimuli, nonresponsive.
- Breathing status: Normal, abnormal, rate abnormalities (>24 or <8), apnea, choking, normal or abnormal chest movement, chest rise and fall, noisy respirations, use of accessory muscles, tripod position, nasal flaring.
- Circulatory status: Radial, carotid pulse, pulse abnormalities, major bleeding, skin color—pink, blue (cyanotic), pale—skin temperature, skin moisture, capillary refill, signs of shock.

Life-threatening conditions must be treated immediately as follows:

- If there is no radial pulse but there is a carotid pulse, lie the patient flat and elevate his or her feet 8 to 12 inches.
- No pulse: Begin CPR.
- Shock: Lay the patient flat, elevate his or her feet 8 to 12 inches, and administer oxygen at 15 L/min.
- Bleeding: Apply pressure to control any bleeding.
- Abnormal breathing: Provide oxygen with a nonrebreather mask. If the patient is unresponsive, cyanotic, or in respiratory distress, use a BVM with supplemental oxygen.
- Unresponsive: Ensure a patent airway.

Conducting a secondary assessment

Following completion of the primary assessment and after attending to any life-threatening problems identified, the EMR should carry out **a secondary assessment** as follows:

- Measure vital signs: Pulse (radial or carotid for adults and brachial for infants and small children), respiration rate, and BP. Using the correct BP cuff size is essential for accuracy. The length of the bladder in the cuff should be equal to 80% of the arm's circumference, and the lower edge of the cuff when positioned should end about one inch above the antecubital fossa (inner elbow). Inflate the cuff to 160 to 180 initially and increase the pressure if pulse sounds are heard at that level.
- Ask further questions as indicated: This may focus on the primary complaint or others, depending on the situation.
- Conduct a physical examination: Examine the body, palpate for areas of tenderness or swelling, and note injuries. Do a brief head-to-toe assessment and compare one side of the body with the other, noting any asymmetry.
- Treat any life-threatening injuries or conditions noted immediately.

Reassessment

Reassessment involves ongoing monitoring of the patient at regular intervals to determine changes in his or her condition or trends such as decreasing BP or increasing agitation. Reassessment is done after a secondary assessment. Unstable patients should be reassessed at least every 5 minutes and stable patients every 15 minutes. Reassessment should include reviewing the primary assessment, taking vital signs, repeating the physical examination (including evaluation of mental status), and monitoring the chief complaint and response to interventions. Reassessment findings should be compared to baseline findings. The patient's airway, ventilation, and circulation should be reassessed as well as the patient's degree of pain—stable, better, or worse. Each intervention should be reassessed for effectiveness and the need for modifications of treatment or if new interventions should be determined. If the patient is receiving oxygen, the tank and all of the equipment should be checked to ensure that they are functioning properly

History taking

History taking should include the following:

- Chief complaint: If the patient is unable to explain, information may be gathered from his or her family, friends, or others who are present. Look for a medical alert bracelet or other such jewelry.
- Nature of the illness or mechanism of injury: Reason for calling EMS, cause of injury, type of illness. Look for environmental clues (fire, drug paraphernalia, motor vehicle accident).
- Signs and symptoms observed or reported by patient: Skin temperature, open wounds, BP abnormalities, pain, or difficulty breathing.
- Precipitating events: Falls, accidents, violence, eating, exercising, walking, driving.
- Pediatric considerations: Check capillary refill to assess blood flow in infants and children younger than 6. Assess the pulse at the brachial artery (inside of the upper arm) for infants to 1 year and the carotid artery in the neck for children older than 1 year of age. May need to use distraction to gain trust and alleviate fear. Encourage parents/caregivers to hold the child if possible and assist in calming the child.
- Geriatric (older adult) considerations: Determine if the patient needs assistive devices, such as hearing aids, eyeglasses, cane, walker, or dentures.

Medicine

Altered mental status

Altered mental status occurs because brain functioning is disrupted. Signs of altered mental status may be subtle (such as slight agitation, lethargy, sleepiness, or forgetfulness) or more obvious (such as disorientation, confusion, personality changes, violent behavior, somnolence, seizures, and coma). An altered mental status may occur abruptly or may have a slower onset, depending on the cause.

- Inadequate oxygenation: Brain cells can only survive about 6 minutes without oxygen, but damage begins to occur after about 60 seconds.
- Inadequate ventilation: Even if oxygen is plentiful, gas exchange is inadequate with impaired ventilation.
- Overdose of medication: May occur with numerous drugs, including opioids/narcotics (such as heroin and oxycodone), antipsychotics, hallucinogens, inhalants, cocaine, methamphetamines, and benzodiazepines.
- Poisoning: Includes arsenic; lead; cyanide; and overdose of medications such as acetaminophen, clonidine, salicylates, calcium channel blockers, and beta blockers.
- Infection: Systemic infections (sepsis), brain abscesses, chronic infections (human immunodeficiency virus/acquired immune deficiency syndrome [HIV/AIDS]).
- Psychological/psychiatric conditions: Includes bipolar disorder, schizophrenia, post-traumatic stress disorder (PTSD), and depression.
- Diabetes: Hyperglycemia and hypoglycemia (especially insulin reaction).

Neurological system

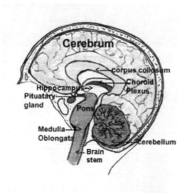

The **neurological (nervous) system** consists of the central nervous system ([CNS] brain, spinal cord, and nerves) and the peripheral nervous system ([PNS] sensory neurons, ganglia [nerve clusters], and nerves connecting to the CNS). The brain consists of the cerebrum (frontal, temporal, parietal, and occipital lobes); the cerebellum; and the brain stem, which is continuous with the spinal cord. The PNS is divided into the autonomic nervous system (ANS) and the somatic nervous system (SoNS). The ANS controls the body's organs and maintains homeostasis (balance). Functions of the ANS include control of the heart rate and function, respiration, digestion, sexual arousal, and other systems. The SoNS comprises cranial and spinal nerves that connect the CNS to the skeletal muscles and skin. The SoNS is the voluntarily controlled component of the PNS, and it receives and responds to external sensory stimuli from the skin and sensory organs.

Ischemic and hemorrhagic strokes

Strokes result from interruption of blood flow to an area of the brain. Ischemic strokes (80%) are caused by blockage of an artery supplying the brain, usually from a thrombus (blood clot) or embolus (traveling clot). Hemorrhagic strokes (20%) result from a ruptured cerebral artery, causing not only a lack of oxygen and nutrients but also edema (swelling) that causes widespread pressure and damage. With both types, patients may experience weakness, paralysis, and loss of sensation in one or more extremities; difficulty speaking or loss of speech; vision impairment; difficulty swallowing; headache; an altered state of consciousness (confusion, disorientation); or coma. Transient ischemic attacks (TIAs) from small clots cause similar but short-lived (minutes to hours) symptoms. Prehospital: Place the patient in the semi-Fowlers or Fowler's position and administer oxygen. The patient may require oral suctioning if the secretions pool. The patient's airway, breathing, and circulation should be assessed. Patients should be transported immediately to the receiving facility because thrombolytic therapy to dissolve blood clots should be administered within 1 to 3 hours.

Seizures

Seizures are sudden, involuntary, abnormal electrical disturbances in the brain that can manifest as alterations of consciousness, spastic tonic and clonic movements, convulsions, and loss of consciousness.

- Tonic-clonic (grand mal): Occurs without warning.
  - Tonic period (10–30 seconds): The eyes roll upward with loss of consciousness, the arms flex, and the body stiffens in symmetric contractions with cyanosis and salivating.
  - Clonic period (usually 30 seconds or longer): Violent rhythmic jerking with contraction and relaxation and sometimes incontinence of urine and feces.

During the seizure, the patient's head and body should be protected from injury, but no attempt should be made to insert anything into the mouth or restrain the patient. If possible, the patient should be screened from spectators and turned onto his or her side (the recovery position) to prevent aspiration. Following seizures, there may be confusion, disorientation, and impairment of motor activity and speech and vision for several hours. Headache, nausea, and vomiting may occur. Prehospital: Monitor the airway, and breathing, and circulation and suction and administer oxygen as needed. Insert an airway for assisted ventilation if the patient is cyanotic.

Partial seizures are caused by an electrical discharge to a localized area of the cerebral cortex, such as the frontal, temporal, or parietal lobes with seizure characteristics related to the area of involvement. They may begin in a focal area and become generalized, often preceded by an aura.

- Simple partial: Unilateral motor symptoms including somatosensory, psychic, and autonomic.
- Aversive: Eyes and head turned away from the focal side.
- Sylvan (usually during sleep): Tonic-clonic movements of the face, salivation, and arrested speech.
- Special sensory: Various sensations (numbness, tingling, prickling, or pain) spreading from one area. May include visual sensations, posturing, or hypertonia. These are rare in patients <8 years.

- Complex (Psychomotor): There is no loss of consciousness, but there may be altered levels of consciousness, and patients may be nonresponsive with amnesia. May involve complex sensorium with bad tastes, auditory or visual hallucinations, a feeling of déjà vu, or strong fear. Patients may carry out repetitive activities, such as walking, running, smacking lips, chewing, or drawling. Patients are rarely aggressive. The seizure is usually followed by prolonged drowsiness and confusion. Occurs from age 3 through adolescence.

Prehospital: Provide supportive care.

Anatomy and physiology of the gastrointestinal (GI) tract

Body part	Function
Mouth	Chews, moistens, begins carbohydrate hydrolysis (the breakdown of food by enzymes), and creates a bolus of food. Connected to the esophagus by the pharynx.
Esophagus	Transports a bolus through the lower esophageal sphincter (which prevents backflow up the esophagus) to the stomach by peristalsis (wavelike contractions).
Stomach	Churns, secretes acids and enzymes, begins hydrolysis of proteins, and creates chyme (a more fluid substance).
Small intestine (about 20 feet long)	Duodenum: Accepts chyme and digests food to prepare for absorption. Jejunum: Absorbs most of the nutrients from the food, including vitamin B_{12}. Accepts bile from the liver and gallbladder to digest fats and pancreatic enzymes from the pancreas to digest proteins, fats, and carbohydrates. Ileum: Contains the ileocecal valve, which controls the flow of chyme into the -large intestine.
Large intestine (about 5 feet long)	Cecum: Reabsorbs fluids and electrolytes. Appendix: Serves no function. Ascending, transverse, descending colon: Reabsorbs water, vitamin K, and electrolytes to form feces.
Rectum	Stores feces.
Anus	Contains sphincters that control the expelling of feces.

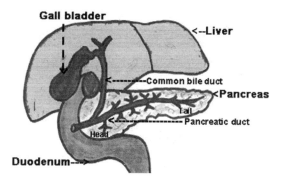

Gastrointestinal (GI) bleeding

Upper **GI bleeding** (mouth to stomach) is characterized by nausea and hematemesis (vomiting of bright-red blood or partially-digested, dark-brown, granulated ["coffee ground"] blood) and/or abdominal pain on palpation. With lower GI bleeding (small intestine to anus), the abdomen may be distended and tender and the patient may be passing blood through the anus. If bleeding has been slow and chronic, the patient may have only vague complaints of weakness and abdominal discomfort. In all cases, blood will mix with the stool. Melena (black-colored stool) usually indicates

- 47 -

an upper GI bleed because the blood has been partially digested. Hematochezia (wine-colored stool or bright-red blood in the stool) indicates a lower GI bleed. Patients develop shock if blood loss is profound (≥40%). Prehospital: Examine the abdomen and note pain; monitor vital signs and note signs of acute blood loss (a fall in BP; an increase in pulse; pallor; or cold, clammy skin). Provide suctioning if needed. Provide supplemental oxygen and ventilation as needed. Place in the recovery position if the patient is vomiting. Place the patient flat with the feet elevated for shock.

Acute abdomen

Acute abdomen is an acute intra-abdominal disorder that occurs with abrupt onset and usually requires emergency surgical intervention, although some patients may respond to other treatments, such as antibiotics. Acute abdomen may result from infection (peritonitis, pancreatitis, cholecystitis, appendicitis, diverticulitis), perforation, rupture of an internal organ (such as the spleen), aortic aneurysm, obstruction, infarction (necrotic tissue resulting from a blood clot or obstructed blood supply). If the blood supply is interrupted, gangrene may occur within 6 hours. Acute abdomen is characterized by inflammation, distension (often including guarding and rigidity), and acute pain (moderate/severe of fewer than 7 days' duration). Abdominal pain is especially concerning in pediatric and geriatric patients and those with impaired immune systems (such as HIV/AIDS patients and those receiving chemotherapy). Acute abdomen in infants and children may indicate conditions not commonly found in adults such as pyloric stenosis, volvulus, and necrotizing enterocolitis. Prehospital: Obtain a medical history regarding the quality, location, and duration of pain as well as referred pain; place the patient in a comfortable position; administer oxygen; and provide rapid transport.

Considerations for pediatric and geriatric patients with abdominal pain

Because **pediatric patients** (infants and small children) have large organs in relation to their size and have very little protection with muscles or bone, organs such as the bladder, liver, and kidneys are more likely to suffer injury from abdominal trauma than adults. The child has a smaller rib cage and pelvic bones, so the abdomen is more vulnerable. Abdominal pain in children may be associated with constipation (right lower quadrant pain) as well as appendicitis, which is characterized by right lower quadrant pain and a lack of appetite, but it may be hard to identify in children because they may not have appreciable or localized pain initially. Pain persisting for ≥48 hours usually indicates a rupture of the appendix. Vomiting and diarrhea may rapidly deplete fluids because of lower fluid volume, resulting in dehydration. **Geriatric patients** with an acute abdomen may not exhibit typical abdominal rigidity or guarding. Additionally, abdominal pain may be an indication of a heart attack rather than a GI problem.

Allergic reactions and anaphylaxis

Allergic reactions are a response of the body's immune system to an antigen (substance), such as peanuts or shellfish. The body produces antibodies (immunoglobulins, such as IgE or non-IgE) that can identify and try to neutralize or destroy antigens. Allergic responses may be mild (local rash, redness, itching, swelling, congestion), moderate (generalized itching, difficulty breathing), or severe (life-threatening anaphylaxis). With **anaphylaxis**, an antigen triggers the release of substances that affect the skin, cardiopulmonary system, and GI system. Histamine causes initial redness and swelling by inducing vasodilation. In some cases, initial reactions may be mild, but subsequent contact can cause a severe, life-threatening response. Symptoms include a sudden onset of weakness, dizziness, and confusion; generalized swelling; itching; severe low BP leading to shock; airway obstruction; nausea and vomiting; hives; diarrhea; seizures; coma; and death. Prehospital: For hypotension and facial swelling, respiratory distress, or swelling of the mouth, provide epinephrine (if authorized) or assist with an autoinjector to the lateral thigh and repeat every 5–10 minutes as needed, provide supplemental oxygen (100%)/ventilation, and transport immediately.

Infectious and contagious diseases

Infectious diseases, which may be communicable or noncommunicable, are those that are caused when microorganisms (such as bacteria, viruses, retroviruses, protozoa, helminths [worms], and fungi) invade the body and cause disease. Noncommunicable diseases may spread from an environmental source, such as contaminated water or food (such as with food poisoning), or from insects that carry the disease (such as with Lyme disease). However, they do not spread from person to person, so only standard precautions are needed when caring for these patients. Contagious diseases are infections that are communicable from person to person. They may be spread through direct physical contact and sneezing or coughing as well as through contact with blood or other body fluids (feces, semen, urine, or perspiration). With contagious diseases, the type of precautions needed depends on the mode of infection, and they may range from contact to droplet to airborne precautions; the type of PPE needed also varies.

Diabetic conditions

Diabetes mellitus is a group of metabolic disorders that involve hyperglycemia (increased blood glucose [sugar]) because of defective production and/or action of insulin. Insulin metabolizes glucose to produce energy as fuel for body cells.

- Type 1: Autoimmune destruction of beta cells in the pancreas results in no or deficient insulin production. Symptoms: Rapid onset, increased thirst, frequent urination, increased hunger, delayed healing, weight loss, frequent infections, and blurred vision.
- Type 2: Insulin baseline may be normal or deficient, but there is no or an inadequate increase in response to a meal, so the glucose level rises but there is decreased uptake by the tissues. Insulin resistance occurs because there is decreased sensitivity to insulin by the tissues. Type 2 diabetes is often related to older age and obesity. Symptoms include slow onset, increased thirst, increased urination, candidal (fungal) infections, delayed healing, and weight gain.
- Gestational: Beta cells in the pancreas are unable to produce adequate insulin during pregnancy, but normal production resumes after delivery. Symptoms include being asymptomatic or having increased thirst and urinary frequency.

Hyperglycemia

Hyperglycemia is high blood glucose (sugar) with a level of greater than 130mg/dL after fasting for 8 hours or greater than 180 mg/dL 2 hours after eating. Hyperglycemia may occur in undiagnosed diabetic patients or in diabetic patients who have taken inadequate insulin; those who have eaten a diet too high in carbohydrates (sugars); or those who are ill, such as with an infection. Initial signs include increased thirst and urination, headaches, lethargy, fatigue, and blurred vision, but if blood glucose is very high (greater than 250 mg/dL), patients may become increasingly somnolent and the patient may develop diabetic ketoacidosis from the buildup of ketones as fat is broken down by the body for energy because glucose cannot be used. The patient may exhibit fruity-smelling breath (from ketones), lapse into a coma, and could die if left untreated. Prehospital: Question the patient about diabetes and the use of diabetic medications. Assist the patient in checking blood sugar level, monitor vital signs, and provide supportive care as needed. Rapid transport is required for altered levels of consciousness.

- 49 -

Hypoglycemia

Hypoglycemia (low blood sugar/glucose) is most often caused by an insulin reaction (too much insulin for the amount of glucose/sugar intake) or an overdose of oral diabetes medications, which stimulate the overproduction of insulin. Hypoglycemia may occur if patients took insulin but skipped a meal, vomited, or exercised too strenuously, depleting the body of sugar/glucose while insulin levels remain high. Increased insulin levels cause glucose levels to fall to at or below 70 mg/dL, initially resulting in tremors, headache, blurred vision, dizziness, and pallor leading to confusion, bizarre behavior, lack of coordination, combative behavior, personality changes, tachycardia, and irregular heartbeat. Severe hypoglycemia may lead to seizures, coma, and death. Hypoglycemia is life threatening if untreated. Infants may have dehydration and seizures; geriatric patients may have dehydration and stroke. Prehospital: Ask the patient about diabetes status and use of diabetes medications. Check the patient's glucose level, and administer oral glucose tablets, one tablespoon of sugar, or a glass of orange juice if the patient is able to swallow; provide rapid transport for altered levels of consciousness.

Age-related considerations with diabetes mellitus

Pediatric patients with diabetes mellitus most commonly have type 1 and are insulin dependent with the peak age for onset during adolescence; however, rates of type 2 diabetes are increasing in young children and adolescents, especially if they are overweight. Children (especially <15) with late stages of hyperglycemia may develop cerebral edema with headache and weakness and changes in mental status, particularly irritability. Children are also more likely to develop hypoglycemia than adults and are more prone to having seizures and becoming dehydrated than adults. Hypoglycemia may result from excessive exercise. Many children may be undiagnosed and may present with diabetic ketoacidosis. **Geriatric patients** often have reduced sensation because of neuropathy associated with diabetes, and they may be unaware of injuries. Geriatric patients are also prone to developing dehydration and infections. Diabetes is the leading cause of lower limb amputation and kidney failure, so many patients on hemodialysis are diabetic. Patients with diabetes may have an atypical presentation of a myocardial infarction (heart attack) without chest pain.

Assessment of psychiatric patients

Assessment of patients with psychological/psychiatric symptoms should begin with a history that includes the patient's age and cultural/spiritual background and whether the patient has experienced similar symptoms previously or has a history of a psychiatric disorder as well as any history of substance abuse. Assessment includes the following:

- General appearance: Note hygiene, grooming, appropriate dress, eye contact, unusual movements (twitching, posturing, repetitive movements), and the appearance and condition of the skin.
- Speech: Note speech cadence and abnormal word use, such as neologisms (invented words), clang associations (rhyming), word salad (string of random words), and associative looseness (ideas shifting from one to another).
- Posture/Gait: Note automatisms (purposeless behaviors, such as drumming fingers), slowed motions, waxy flexibility (maintaining an awkward position for extended periods of time), ability to walk, and abnormalities of gait.
- Mental status: Note the patient's state of being alert versus nonalert, responsive versus nonresponsive, and coherent versus noncoherent; clarity of ideas; suicidal ideation; and desire for self-harm.

- Mood and affect: Note facial expressions, expressed emotions, and affect (blunted, broad, flat, inappropriate, restricted).
- Memory/Intellectual processes: Note if memory and intellectual processes are intact or impaired. Is the patient disoriented and confused or alert and responsive?
- Attention: Note if the patient's attention is focused or unfocused.

Behavioral alterations

Behavioral alterations may include agitation, anger, throwing temper tantrums (children), acting aggressively (adolescents/adult), exhibiting poor judgment, and acting inappropriately. Behavioral alterations may result from psychiatric disorders (such as depression, schizophrenia, and bipolar disorder) and psychiatric medications, as well as numerous other causes, including the following:

- Hypoglycemia/Low blood sugar (insulin reaction).
- Lack of adequate oxygen interferes with brain function.
- Shock (low BP; a rapid pulse results in inadequate blood supply to the brain).
- Mind-altering substances (cocaine, methamphetamine, lysergic acid diethylamide [LSD], Rohypnol [the date-rape drug]).
- Brain infection (meningitis, encephalitis, brain abscess).
- Seizure disorders (epilepsy, other causes of seizures).
- Poisoning/Overdose (lead poisoning, drug overdose).
- Malnutrition resulting in inadequate nourishment of brain tissue.
- Substance abuse (drug or alcohol abuse/withdrawal).
- Heat extremes (hypothermia/hyperthermia).

Indications of being a danger to self or others include severe agitation, hallucinations, delusional thinking, paranoia, self-destructive behavior (cutting, drug/alcohol abuse, promiscuity, risk-taking activities), depression, and suicide attempts. A patient may pose a risk to others if he or she is behaving in a threatening or violent manner and has a weapon (club, gun, knife, baseball bat).

Assessing for risk of suicide

Suicidal ideation occurs frequently in those with mood disorders or depression (common in geriatric patients). Although females are more likely to attempt suicide, males actually successfully commit suicide three times more often than females, primarily because females tend to take overdoses from which they can be revived whereas males choose more violent means (jumping from a high place, shooting, or hanging). This holds true for adolescents and adults. Risk factors include psychiatric disorders (schizophrenia, bipolar disorder, post-traumatic stress disorder [PTSD], and substance abuse), physical disorders (HIV/AIDS, diabetes, traumatic brain injury, spinal cord injury), and social problems (bullying). Passive suicidal ideation involves wishing to be dead or thinking about dying without making plans, whereas active suicidal ideation involves making plans. Patients at risk should be questioned about their feelings, problems, plans for suicide, and access to weapons. High-risk findings include the following:

- Violent suicide attempt (knives, guns) or access to a weapon.
- History of a suicide attempt and a suicide attempt with a low chance of rescue.
- Ongoing psychosis or disordered thinking.
- Ongoing severe depression and feelings of helplessness.
- Lack of a social support system.

Methods to calm patients with behavioral emergencies

Patients with **behavioral emergencies** are often agitated and may be confused, fearful and/or aggressive, so the EMR must remain calm and approach the patient slowly; remain at a safe distance; and avoid fast movements, threatening postures, or attempts at physical contact, acknowledging the patient's agitation and offering assistance ("I can see that you're upset, and I want to help") and maintaining eye contact (unless the person is violent and reacts aggressively). The EMR should encourage the patient to talk about what is causing the behavior and should answer questions honestly while avoiding threatening, arguing, or challenging the patient. If the patient is suffering hallucinations or delusional thinking, the EMR should avoid playing along ("I don't see what you do") but should also avoid contradicting the patient directly when responding. Family or friends may assist with intervention. The EMR should not leave the patient unattended and should try to lower distressing stimuli (such as lights and noise) and consider contacting law enforcement. Restraints should be avoided if possible.

Circulatory system

The **circulatory system** controls blood flow throughout the body and to the tissues, controls gas exchange (carbon dioxide and oxygen), serves as a reservoir for blood, maintains blood pH through a buffer system, responds to infections, and facilitates coagulation (blood clotting). The circulatory system includes the cardiovascular system (heart and blood vessels) and the blood.

- Heart: Has four chambers, upper (right atrium and left atrium) and lower (right ventricle and left ventricle). The heart muscle receives blood from two major coronary arteries and their branches.
- Blood vessels: The venous system includes the veins, venules, and venous capillaries, and it brings blood back to the heart via the inferior and superior vena cava. The arterial system, including the coronary arteries, branches from the aorta after it leaves the heart and includes arteries, arterioles, and arterial capillaries.
- Blood: Red blood cells (erythrocytes); white blood cells (leukocytes including monocytes, lymphocytes, basophils, neutrophils, and eosinophils); platelets (thrombocytes); and plasma, the liquid portion of the blood (which contains clotting factors).

The circulatory system is responsible for the oxygenation of cells, perfusion (carrying blood with oxygen, glucose, and nutrients to cells), and removing waste products such as carbon dioxide.

Chest pain

Chest pain may indicate angina (pain from temporary constriction/blockage of blood flow in the coronary arteries) or a heart attack (pain caused by blockage of blood flow to the heart muscle because of a blood clot [most common] or hemorrhage, resulting in the death of heart tissue). Heart problems in children are often associated with congenital heart disease. Geriatric patients may not have chest pain with a heart attack. Make note of the following:

- Character, location, and severity of the pain.
- Radiation of pain, to the neck, jaw, arms, back, jaw, and/or stomach.
- Shortness of breath at rest or with exertion or worsening when lying flat.
- Skin: Cold, clammy skin is common with a heart attack.
- Vital signs: Note BP, pulse (rapid, irregular, slow), and respirations.
- Other: Note nausea and/or vomiting and dizziness/lightheadedness.

Prehospital: Provide the patient with a position of comfort (often semi-Fowler's if there is shortness of breath), provide a high concentration of oxygen with a nonrebreather mask, and question the patient about medications taken recently and/or medications taken for pain (such as aspirin or nitroglycerin), and provide rapid transport.

Management of a patient with chest pain begins with providing support and reassurance because patients are often very frightened. The patient should be placed in a position of comfort, usually the semi-Fowler's position, especially if he or she is experiencing shortness of breath, and vital signs (blood pressure [BP], pulse [P], and respiration rate [R]) should be monitored. The patient should be encouraged to rest. Respiratory compromise may require supplemental high-concentration oxygen with a nonrebreather mask. The patient should be questioned about taking the following medications and, if so, the dosage and time should be noted:

- Aspirin (for suspected heart attack; Bayer, Heartline, ZORprin, Empirin): Provide 162 to 325 mg chewable (preferred). Contraindicated with GI bleeding, stroke.
- Nitroglycerin (for suspected angina; Nitro-Dur, Nitrolingual, NitroMist): Provide 0.4 mg sublingually repeated every 3–5 minutes up to three doses. Contraindicated if the patient has recently taken Viagra, had a stroke, or has excessive bleeding.
- Oral glucose (for suspected hypoglycemia/insulin reaction): Glucose tablets, solution.

All patients with chest pain should be transported because even mild chest discomfort may indicate that the patient is having a heart attack, especially in older patients and female patients, who often have atypical symptoms.

Carbon monoxide poisoning

Carbon monoxide poisoning occurs when people breathe in carbon monoxide, usually related to industrial or household accidents or suicide attempts. Carbon monoxide binds to hemoglobin 200 times more readily than oxygen, and once the carbon monoxide binds to hemoglobin (creating carboxyhemoglobin), the hemoglobin can no longer bind to or transport oxygen, resulting in hypoxemia (low blood oxygen). Symptoms vary depending on the percentage of saturation. At 10%, patients may complain of headache and nausea. At >20%, a patient becomes increasingly weak and confused with alterations in mental status. At >30%, a patient may have dyspnea, chest pain, and increased confusion. When the level continues to increase, a patient may experience seizures, coma, and death. The patient's skin color may be cyanotic, pink, or bright cherry red (but this is not a reliable sign). Prehospital: Manage the patient's airway/ventilation/oxygen supplementation with 100% oxygen with a nonrebreather mask. Note: Pulse oximetry cannot distinguish carbon monoxide from oxygen.

Poisoning by nerve agents/cholinergics

Nerve agents/Cholinergics are toxic chemicals (organophosphates) that damage the nervous system and bodily functions, leading to death in a short time. Nerve agents include tabun (GA), sarin (GB), soman (GD), and VX, and they are used in terrorist attacks. GA, BG, and GD persist in the environment for 10 minutes to 24 hours during summer and 2 hours to 3 days during winter (cold weather) and have very fast action. VX persists longer in the environment and is more lethal. Symptoms of exposure (gas/aerosol) include SLUDGE (salivation, lacrimation, urination, defecation, GI upset, and emesis), runny nose, pupil contraction, vision impairment, slurred speech, chest pain, hallucinations, respiratory distress, and coma. High doses may cause immediate seizures and death. Prehospital: Move away from the area quickly or shelter in place, remove all clothing, and wash the patient's body with large amounts of soap and water. Use an autoinjector for atropine and pralidoxime (separate injections [Mark I] or combined dose [DuoDote]) unless there is only mild tearing or a runny nose, and use diazepam for seizures. Provide airway/ventilation/oxygenation and circulation support.

Poison control resources

The **National Capital Poison Center** provides a website with an online tool—webPOISONCONTROL—(https://triage.webpoisoncontrol.org/#/exclusions) and a telephone number (1-800-222-1222) for people who swallow (ingest) or come into contact (absorbed, inhaled, injected) with poisonous (toxic) substances.

- webPOISONCONTROL: Can be used for patients (ages 6 months to 79 years and nonpregnant women) who are asymptomatic and unintentionally swallowed a single drug or medication, household product, or berries over a short period of time (minutes to a few hours) and are otherwise healthy.
- Telephone contact: For all other situations, including a patient with symptoms, pregnant women, nonswallowing contact, those ages <6 months or >79, or those who swallowed materials or substances other than those listed online assistance. Telephone contact can be made for any poisoning if it is preferred to online assistance.

This service is free and usually requires about 3 minutes for a response. When calling, be prepared to describe the substance (include the product name and dosage for medications), amount swallowed, age of patient, weight of patient, time since exposure, and the patient's ZIP Code and email address. If unsure of the amount of the poison or the weight of the patient, estimates are acceptable.

Safe use and disposal of autoinjectors

Autoinjectors are spring-loaded syringe/needle devices that contain preloaded doses of medication and can be easily administered by following the directions on the devices. Autoinjectors are available for nerve agent treatment for emergency medical personnel—Mark I and DuoDote.

- Atropine autoinjector: For symptoms of nerve damage (increases heart rate, dries secretions, dilates pupils, and reduces GI upset).
- Pralidoxime (2-PAM chloride) autoinjector: For symptoms of nerve damage, twitching, and difficulty breathing.
- Diazepam autoinjector: For convulsions associated with nerve agents.

Wear appropriate PPE, remove the safety cap, cleanse the skin with alcohol, and (holding the device perpendicular to the skin) apply firm pressure with the tip of the injector against the skin in the

- 54 -

outer thigh until the device fires the needle into the muscle tissue (avoid jabbing). Then, hold the autoinjector in place for at least 10 seconds to ensure that the medication is completely injected. Carefully remove the needle from the skin. Avoid touching the needle, and do not attempt to recap it. Dispose of the intact device in a sharps container.

Age-related concerns related to toxicology

Age-related concerns related to **toxicolog**y include the following:

- Toddlers are at risk of ingestion of toxic substances because their taste buds are not yet fully developed and this allows them to drink foul-tasting substances, such as cleaning supplies, which may be kept under a sink where a child has easy access if the cabinet is not secured. Household substances that pose a substantial risk include perfumes, cosmetics, and alcohol. Toddlers may also ingest unsecured medications.
- Adolescents, who often experiment with drugs and alcohol, are at risk from alcohol poisoning and overdose or severe reaction to illicit drugs. Additionally, adolescents often attempt suicide with acetaminophen (Tylenol), sometimes to gain attention, without realizing that it can cause liver failure and death, even after resuscitation.
- Geriatric patients are most at risk from medication errors, such as taking the wrong medication, taking medications belonging to friends or family, or taking the wrong dose of a medication.

Hemodialysis

Hemodialysis is used primarily for those who have progressed from renal insufficiency to uremia with end-stage renal (kidney) disease (ESRD). With hemodialysis, blood is circulated outside of the body through a dialyzer (a synthetic semipermeable membrane), which filters the blood and removes waste products and excess fluids. A vascular access device, such as a catheter, fistula, or graft, must be established for hemodialysis, with fistulas and grafts usually being placed in an arm and a catheter being placed in the upper chest (into the superior vena cava). Tubing from the dialysis machine attaches to the access device for treatments, which are usually done for 4 hours three times weekly. Emergent conditions include low BP, nausea/vomiting, irregular pulse, cardiac arrest, bleeding from the access site, and difficulty breathing. Prehospital: Manage the patient's airway/ventilation/oxygen supplementation, apply pressure to stop any bleeding, position the patient flat if he or she is in shock and upright if having difficulty breathing.

Vaginal bleeding

Vaginal bleeding may indicate heavy menstrual bleeding (menorrhagia) or abnormal bleeding between cycles (metrorrhagia). Vaginal bleeding may also be an indication of ectopic pregnancy or spontaneous abortion; in postmenopausal women, it may be a sign of endometrial cancer. Menorrhagia may be caused by hormonal imbalance, clotting disorders, uterine fibroids, and endometrial polyps. Metrorrhagia may be caused by infection, cancer, and cervical/endometrial polyps. Symptoms may include cramping and abdominal pain, depending on the cause. It's important to determine when the bleeding started and about how much blood had been lost (the number of sanitary pads that are saturated per hour, for example) as well as the presence or absence of pain. If blood loss is excessive, the patient may exhibit signs of shock. Prehospital: Use standard precautions, manage the patient's airway, ventilate, and provide oxygen as needed. Monitor vital signs. Position the patient flat for shock.

Nosebleed (epistaxis)

Recurrent **nosebleed (epistaxis)** is common in young children (ages 2–10), especially boys, and it is often related to nose picking, dry climate, trauma, or central heating. Incidence also increases between 50–80 years of age and may be associated with nonsteroidal anti-inflammatory drugs (NSAIDs), hypertension, and anticoagulants. Patients abusing cocaine may suffer nosebleeds because of damage to the mucosa. The anterior (front) nares have plentiful blood vessels and bleed easily, usually from one nostril. Bleeding in the posterior (back) nares is more dangerous and can result in considerable blood loss. Blood may flow through both nostrils or backward into the throat, and the person may be observed swallowing and may vomit blood. The blood may block the airway in unconscious patients. Prehospital: Sit the patient in an upright position, leaning forward so the blood doesn't flow down the throat if the patient is conscious; pinch the nostrils together firmly for at least 10 minutes; and advise the patient to avoid sniffing or blowing the nose.

Shock and Resuscitation

Shock

Shock is a life-threatening condition that occurs when the tissues do not receive adequate oxygen, such as with severe bleeding or fluid loss, severe infection, heart failure, or abnormal dilation of the blood vessels. Indications of shock include extreme thirst; anxiety and restlessness; weak, rapid pulse; altered mental status progressing to loss of consciousness; rapid, shallow respirations; hypotension (low BP—often a late sign); and cool, clammy, pale skin with mottling sometimes on extremities from inadequate perfusion. If left untreated, shock may lead to cardiac arrest. Note that geriatric patients may have a higher baseline respiration and heart rate and irregular pulse. Prehospital: Request the assistance of advanced EMS if necessary, apply pressure to control bleeding, perform spinal stabilization if needed, place the patient in the shock position (flat with feet elevated above the level of the heart, 8 to 12 inches), manage the patient's airway/ventilation and administer high-concentration oxygen, provide warming blankets to maintain body temperature, apply a pneumatic antishock garment per protocol if available, and provide reassurance. Provide rapid transport if needed.

Respiratory failure/arrest

Respiratory failure occurs when ventilation is insufficient for adequate gas exchange so that levels of carbon dioxide in the blood increase and levels of oxygen decreases. Respiratory failure may result from respiratory infection (pneumonia, tuberculosis), heart failure, chronic respiratory illness (asthma, chronic bronchitis, COPD), trauma, and depression of the central nervous system (usually from medications or trauma). Respiratory failure may be acute with sudden onset or chronic, developing over time. If untreated, respiratory failure can lead to **respiratory arrest**, which in turn leads to cardiac arrest. Indications of respiratory failure include altered mental status, cyanosis, labored breathing (dyspnea and orthopnea), coughing, fatigue, diminished breath sounds, and the presence of rales (crackles) and rhonchi (a snoring/whistling sound). Patients may have hemoptysis (bloody sputum). The patient's oxygen saturation level is lower than 90% per pulse oximeter. Prehospital: Manage the patient's airway/ventilation/oxygen supplementation. Positive-pressure ventilation may be needed. Place the patient in a position of comfort (usually high Fowler's).

Cardiopulmonary resuscitation (CPR) for cardiac arrest

Cardiac arrest of unknown cause in adults or children is usually treated as though it were ventricular fibrillation or pulseless ventricular tachycardia, but the protocol varies. **Cardiopulmonary resuscitation (CPR)** involves the following components:

- Immediate defibrillation (one shock) is performed according to protocol with an AED/manual defibrillator (preferred) followed by CPR, beginning with compressions (30:2 compression to ventilation at the rate of 100–120 per minute at least 2 inches deep; two-finger compressions to one-third of the chest depth for infants and children) for 2 minutes/5 cycles and repeat defibrillation.
- Repeat cycles of 2 minutes CPR and defibrillation. (Laypeople use compression-only CPR.)

- If a defibrillator is not readily available, CPR may begin first. Note that if a BVM is used, the break in compressions should not exceed 10 seconds. If an advanced airway/intubation is in place, ventilation should be at the rate of 8 to 10 per minutes, maintaining oxygen saturation ≥94% but <100% with ventilation between compressions.
- The $ETCO_2$ value should be 10–20 mm Hg if chest compressions are adequate, increasing to 35 to 45 mm Hg with return of spontaneous circulation (ROSC).

Ethical issues in withholding resuscitation attempts

Although the goal of EMS is to save lives, it is not always possible or ethical to carry out resuscitation efforts. **Withholding resuscitation** is justified under the following conditions:

- The patient's condition is not compatible with life (massive injuries, decapitation, crushed chest, severe open head injury with loss of brain tissue), and the patient is not breathing and has no pulse.
- The patient exhibits obvious signs of death, such as rigor mortis or livor mortis, indicating that he or she can no longer be resuscitated.
- The patient has a do-not-resuscitate (DNR) form available, and it is properly signed. Note: The EMR cannot accept the word of family or friends that the patient does not want to be resuscitated without a DNR order.
- Conditions are unsafe to approach the patient and/or administer resuscitation efforts. This may occur, for example, if there are gunshots heard in the area, if the patient is pinned under a motor vehicle, or if the patient cannot safely be reached in time because of difficult terrain.

Emergency defibrillation with an automated external defibrillator (AED)

Emergency defibrillation is done for acute ventricular fibrillation or ventricular tachycardia with no audible or palpable pulse; it is ineffective for asystole or pulseless electrical activity. Defibrillation delivers an electrical discharge through paddles applied to both sides of the chest. **Automated external defibrillators (AEDs)** are frequently used by first responders, although manual defibrillators require less downtime from CPR. The procedure is as follows:

- Turn on the AED.
- Apply pads to the chest (the position may vary according to the manufacturer). Infants and small children: If pads may touch, apply one to the chest and one to the back.
- Plug in the connector if necessary.
- Do not touch the patient while the AED analyzes the heart rhythm.
- Follow the directions for shocking, and warn others to stand clear.
- Continue CPR, beginning with compressions for 2 minutes/five cycles between defibrillations.

If the patient is wet, wipe off his or her chest before applying the pads. Remove any transdermal patches on the chest, and shave excessive hair before applying the pads. If the patient has an implanted device, the pads should be placed at least 1 inch (2.5 cm) away.

Techniques of the Heimlich maneuver for choking

The universal sign of choking is when a person clutches his or her throat and appears to be choking or gasping for breath. If the person can speak ("Can you speak?") or cough, the **Heimlich maneuver** is not usually necessary. The Heimlich maneuver can be done with the victim sitting, standing, or supine.

The Heimlich procedure for children (≥1 year) and adults is as follows:

- Wrap your arms around the victim's waist from the back if sitting or standing. Make a fist and place the thumb side against the victim's abdomen slightly above the umbilicus. Grasp this hand with the other and thrust sharply upward to force air out of the lungs.
- Repeat as needed.
- If the victim loses consciousness, ease him or her into a supine position on the floor, place your hands similarly to CPR but over the abdomen while sitting astride the victim's legs. Repeat upward compressions five times. If no ventilation occurs, attempt to sweep the mouth and ventilate the lungs mouth to mouth. Repeat compressions and ventilations until recovery.

Indications of choking in infants of less than 1 year include lack of breathing, gasping, cyanosis, and inability to cry. The procedures for **Heimlich chest thrusts** includes the following:

- Position the infant in the prone (face-down) position along your forearm with the infant's head being lower than the trunk, being sure to support the head so the airway is not blocked.
- Using the heel of the hand, deliver five forceful upward blows between the shoulder blades.
- Sandwich the child between your two arms, and turn the infant into the supine position and drape over your thigh with the head lower than the trunk and the head being supported.
- Using two fingers (as for CPR compressions), give up to five thrusts (about 1.5 inches deep) to the lower third of the sternum.
- Only do a finger sweep and remove a foreign object if the object is visible. Repeat five back blows, five chest thrusts until the foreign body is ejected.
- If the infant loses consciousness, begin CPR. If a pulse is noted but spontaneous respirations are absent, continue with ventilation only.

Trauma

Characteristics of different types of bleeding

Types of bleeding	Characteristics	Prehospital
Arterial	Bright-red spurting blood that is difficult to control; it lessens as the BP falls.	Using standard precautions and PPE as indicated, apply sterile gauze dressing and pressure with fingertips if it is a small bleed or apply direct hand pressure if it is more copious. As dressings saturate, add new dressings but don't remove the old ones. Keep the patient in the shock position, especially with an arterial bleed or severe blood loss, and keep him or her warm. Avoid giving food or fluids and transport immediately for severe bleeding or suspected
Venous	Dark-red blood flowing in a steady stream; it may be copious, but it is easier to control than an arterial bleed.	
Capillary	Oozing; it usually clots spontaneously.	

Sucking chest wounds and chest impalements

Type	Characteristics	Prehospital
Sucking	This is an open pneumothorax in which air sucks into the thoracic cavity, deflating the lung, usually through a penny-size or larger wound. Patients will exhibit respiratory distress, absent breath sounds on the affected side, wound gurgling on inspiration, and bubbling of blood about the wound.	Apply an occlusive dressing with an Asherman Chest Seal dressing or with Vaseline gauze covered with secured (taped on three sides) plastic wrap or aluminum foil and place the patient in a position of comfort.
Impalement	This is a penetrating wound with an object impaled into the chest. Symptoms may be similar to those listed above depending on the site of impalement and the depth.	Expose the wound area, and secure the object manually with a bulky dressing. Do not remove the object unless it is necessary for performing chest compressions (CPR). Control the bleeding.

Eviscerations and impaled objects

Eviscerations occur with open abdominal wounds, such as opening incisions or traumatic injuries, which allow the internal organs (often the intestines) to protrude externally. Surgical repair is required to reinsert the organs into the abdomen. The patient may go into shock, especially if the evisceration is part of other major injuries (common in trauma cases). Prehospital: Provide supportive care, cover the eviscerated organs with thick sterile gauze dressings moistened with normal saline (NS) but do not attempt to reinsert the organs, manage the patient's airway/ventilation/oxygen supplementation as needed, provide rapid transport. **Impalements** occur when an object penetrates the abdomen and remains in place and may be associated with multiple internal injuries and bleeding. Prehospital: Do not remove the object, but expose the abdomen and manually secure the object with bulky dressings, and control bleeding. Prehospital: Provide supportive care, manage the patient's airway/ventilation/oxygen supplementation as needed, and provide rapid transport.

Orthopedic trauma

Fractures usually result from trauma (falls, auto accidents), but <u>pathologic fractures</u> can result from minor force to diseased bones (osteoporosis or cancerous lesions). <u>Stress fractures</u> are caused by repetitive trauma (forced marching). <u>Salter-Harris fractures</u> involve the cartilaginous epiphyseal plate near the ends of long bones in children who are growing, and this can impair bone growth. Fracture types are listed as follows:

- Open fractures with soft-tissue injury and a break in the skin overlying the fracture, including puncture wounds from external forces or bone fragments; these can result in osteomyelitis (bone infection).
- Closed fractures involve a broken bone but no break in the skin.

Symptoms include pain, deformity or angulation, swelling, bruising, inability to move the joint or bear weight, grating on movement, and impaired function or circulation. Isolated fractures are usually not life threatening, but pelvic and femur fractures may involve severe blood loss. Prehospital: Cover open wounds with sterile dressings, manually stabilize and immobilize the fracture area but do not replace protruding bones, apply a cold pack, place the patient in a position of comfort.

Subluxation (partial dislocation of a joint) and **luxation** (complete dislocation) can cause neurovascular compromise, which can be permanent if reduction is delayed. This is especially a problem with <u>hip dislocations</u>, which most commonly occur in automobile accidents when the person's knees impact the dashboard. <u>Elbow dislocations</u> often result from athletic injuries and may cause nerve damage. <u>Shoulder dislocations</u> are the most common type and also often result from athletic injuries. They may become chronic. <u>Knee dislocations</u> may result in severe injury to the popliteal artery, and this can lead to amputation, so rapid transport and emergent surgical repair are indicated. Differentiating between fractures and dislocations can be difficult because the symptoms and appearance are often similar. A deformity may not be evident, or it may be obscured by edema, or edema may give the appearance of a deformity. Extensive bruising may occur with all types of injuries, and pain may occur even with minor soft-tissue injuries. Prehospital: Splint and immobilize the area, apply a cold compress, and place the patient in a position of comfort.

Amputations may be partial or complete and result from crush, guillotine (cutting), or avulsion (twisting) injuries. A <u>simple amputation</u> requires no extrication and other injuries or shock are absent, but a <u>complex amputation</u> may involve multiple injuries, shock, and delayed treatment because of extrication. The amputated limb should be treated initially as though it could be reattached, although single digits (except the thumb) and lower limbs are not usually reattached. The part should be irrigated with normal saline (NS) to remove debris; wrapped in NS-moistened gauze; and placed in a sealed plastic bag, which should be immersed in ice water. The body part should not freeze and should not be placed directly on ice. Prehospital: Manage the patient's airway/ventilation/oxygen supplementation; control bleeding by using direct pressure or, if there is severe hemorrhage, by applying a BP cuff proximal to (above) the injury 70 mm Hg greater than the systolic BP for <30 minutes; irrigate the stump with NS if it is dirty; cover the open area with NS-moistened gauze; and elevate the stump.

Soft-tissue injuries

Injury	Characteristics	Prehospital
Abrasion	Painful, superficial scraping of the outermost layer of skin. Little or no bleeding.	Irrigate with water or NS to remove debris and cover with a nonadherent dressing.
Laceration	Cut or break in skin from an impact with a sharp object. Bleeding may vary from mild to severe.	Apply pressure to control bleeding; irrigate to remove debris if necessary; and cover with dry, sterile gauze dressing.
Puncture	Wound from an impact with a sharp, pointed object (knife, bullet), which may exhibit little external bleeding but major internal bleeding and soft-tissue damage. An exit wound may be present.	Apply pressure to control bleeding, manage the patient's airway/ventilation/oxygen supplementation, and provide rapid transport if the patient is unstable.
Impaled object	Penetrating object remains in the wound.	Leave the object in place and pad with bulky dressings.
Foreign body in the eye(s)	Patient has pain, tearing, redness, blurred or impaired vision from dirt, dust, chemical, or other material in the eye(s).	Cover both eyes loosely (avoiding pressure) to prevent movement. If the contamination is from a chemical, flush with copious amounts of NS or water.

Burn injuries and the rule of nines

Burn injuries may be chemical, electrical, or thermal and are assessed by the area affected, percentage of the body burned, and the depth of the burn, as follows:

- First-degree burns are superficial and affect the epidermis, causing erythema and pain.
- Second-degree burns extend through the dermis (partial thickness), resulting in blistering and sloughing of epidermis.
- Third-degree burns affect the underlying tissue, including the vasculature, muscles, and nerves (full thickness).

Burns are classified according to the American Burn Association's criteria as follows:

- Minor: <10% body surface area (BSA) or 2% BSA with third-degree burns without serious risk to the face, hands, feet, or perineum.
- Moderate: 10%–20% BSA combined second- and third-degree burns in adult; age <10 years or ≤10% third-degree without serious risk to the face, hands, feet, or perineum.
- Major: 20% BSA; ≥10% third-degree burns; all burns are to the face, hands, feet, or perineum and will result in functional/cosmetic defect; or burns with inhalation or other major trauma.

The rule of nines estimates the BSA burned: Adults—head 9%, trunk (front) 18%, trunk (back) 18%, arm 9%, leg 18%, perineum 1%. Infants/Children—head 18%, trunk (front) 18%, trunk (back) 18%, arm 9%, leg 13.5%, perineum 1%.

Management of burns

Those with severe burns may develop shock and impairment of all major body systems. If the burning process is ongoing (smoldering clothes, tissue), room-temperature water or NS should be applied to stop the burning and any smoldering clothes or jewelry should be removed, although if the clothing is adhered to the skin, it should be left in place. Facial or airway burns are a major concern, so the airway must be monitored constantly with interventions as necessary. The burned area should be covered with clean, dry dressings, and the patient should be kept warm for transport. Children experience greater fluid and heat loss because of their greater body surface area relative to their size, and the EMR should be alert to the possibility of child abuse. With **chemical burns**, any dry powder should be brushed off and wet chemicals should be flushed with copious amounts of water (by an EMR wearing gloves and eye protection). With **electrical burns**, internal burns may be more severe than external burns, and the patient is at risk of cardiac arrest.

Dressings and bandages

Dressing/Bandage	Characteristics
Sterile gauze	4×4 (sponge) or roller/wrapping gauze (Kerlix) that is used to protect skin or pack wounds to control bleeding. Roller gauze may be used to secure other dressings.
Nonadherent dressings	Designed not to stick to open wounds because of their special coating (Teflon, foam, petrolatum, hydrogel). Used on abrasions, burns, and lightly draining wounds.
Occlusive dressings	These have a waxy coating to make an air- and water-tight seal, but they are not as absorbent as gauze. Used for sucking chest wounds, abdominal eviscerations, and lacerations of the external jugular vein or carotid.
Trauma dressings	Dressings that often include a nonadherent pad, clotting agent embedded in the dressing, and an elastic wrap in one piece so that it can be rapidly applied (such as an ACE bandage); they include QuikClot Combat Gauze and Celox Rapid hemostatic gauze. Especially useful to control bleeding and apply pressure to a wound.
Adhesive, roller bandages	May be elastic or nonelastic, and they are used to secure other dressings and/or apply compression.

Head and spine injuries

Injury	Characteristics	Prehospital
Head	Open: Bleeding. Closed: Swelling and bruising, may have depression of the skull. May have an underlying injury.	Apply direct pressure to control the bleeding; apply dry, sterile dressings. Monitor the patient's mental status.
Scalp	Copious bleeding may occur. May cause shock in infants and young children.	As above. Manage the patient's airway/ventilation/oxygen supplementation if needed. Rapid transport is required with shock.
Brain	Direct injury to brain tissue or damage from bleeding inside the skull may occur. Altered mental status.	As above. Rapid transport is required.

Spine	Suspect with motor vehicle/pedestrian accidents; falls; hanging; blunt or penetrating trauma to head, neck or torso; diving accidents; and unresponsive trauma patients. May have tenderness in the area; pain on moving; numbness, tingling, or weakness; inability to feel or move below the injury; difficulty breathing; incontinence (bowel and/or bladder).	Responsive: Manually stabilize the patient's head and neck in the position he or she is found until a cervical collar and backboard are in place; question pain, sensations, and the ability to move. Unresponsive: Stabilize the head and neck as above; manage the patient's airway, ventilation, oxygen supplementation; and question witnesses. Rapid transport.

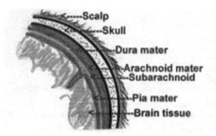

Trauma

Pediatric trauma

Note the pediatric assessment triangle (appearance, work of breathing, and circulation). Respiration rates vary with age, but the use of accessory muscles and sternal retraction indicate respiratory distress. Assess the brachial pulse in infants—a slow pulse indicates hypoxia. Trauma is the leading cause of death in pediatric patients, and hypoventilation is the leading cause of cardiac arrest. BP values are not reliable for small children, who may have normal BP in compensated shock. Shaken baby syndrome should be considered with pediatric trauma; it is believed to be the result of vigorous shaking of an infant, causing acute subdural hematoma (brain hemorrhage) and retinal (eye) hemorrhages. It is believed that the shaking of the brain causes coup (front) and contrecoup (back) damage as well as damaging the vessels and nerves with resultant cerebral edema (swelling). Prehospital: Manage hypovolemia/shock, prevent hypothermia, and manage the patient's airway/ventilation/oxygen supplementation as needed. Ventilate if the patient is bradycardic. BVM ventilation is usually the best ventilation method for children.

Pregnancy trauma

The mother and fetus are each considered to be patients. Trauma is the cause of 46% of maternal deaths, and blunt trauma is the cause of up to 38% of fetal deaths. Pregnant patients are susceptible to falls (especially in the third trimester when the mother's center of gravity shifts) and domestic abuse (which may include blunt trauma and penetrating trauma from knife or gunshot wounds). However, most trauma in pregnant women occurs as the result of motor vehicle accidents. Pregnant women have an increased blood volume and heart rate, impaired venous return if in a supine (flat) position in the third trimester, and increased risk of vomiting and aspiration.

Hypovolemia/shock reduces the amount of oxygen going to the fetus, resulting in fetal stress. Vaginal bleeding may occur. Prehospital: Have suction available, monitor the airway/ventilation/oxygenation and provide 100% oxygen per nonrebreather mask and ventilation assistance if needed (especially with symptoms of shock), transport on the left side (tilt the immobilization board if necessary), and provide rapid transport.

Geriatric trauma

These patients are more susceptible to trauma because of aging processes, and they may be less able to maintain normal vital signs during hemorrhage. About 80% of patients older than age 65 have one chronic illness, and 50% have two. Polypharmacy is common, and medications may affect vital signs and blood clotting. Response times may be slower than normal. Falls are the most common cause of injury in geriatric patients. Elder abuse should be suspected if patients have repeated injuries. Scalding is the most common burn injury and is often deeper because of thinning skin. The risk of cerebral bleeding with trauma is increased because of brain shrinkage. The cough reflex may be lessened. Fractures are common because of osteoporosis, especially hip fractures. Prehospital: Splint fractures, monitor the airway/ventilation/oxygen supplementation, monitor oxygenation with pulse oximetry, suction if necessary, and check the mouth for dentures (which may obstruct the airway). Note: Spinal curvature may require padding of the spinal board.

Trauma in cognitively impaired patients

Disorders may include Alzheimer's or other forms of dementia, traumatic brain injuries, strokes, Down's syndrome, and autistic spectrum disorders, so patients may be of all ages. Patients may be more at risk of trauma, and assessment and history taking may be difficult. Perceptions of pain may be altered, and psychological reactions may vary. Patients who are cognitively impaired are often more vulnerable to physical, sexual, and psychological abuse and may be unable to or afraid to report abuse. Patients may have an exaggerated response to pain or injury and may be very frightened and agitated or withdrawn, so the extent of injury may be difficult to determine. Prehospital: Remain supportive, reassure the patient, avoid any use of medical jargon, and use simple statements (asking one question at a time), use yes/no questions, obtain information from the caregiver if necessary, and treat as indicated by the patient's condition.

Generalized hypothermia

Generalized hypothermia occurs when the body temperature falls to below-normal levels.

- Mild: 32°C–35°C (89.6°F–95°F).
- Moderate: 28°C–32°C (82.4°F–95°F).
- Severe: <32°C (<82.4°F).

Contributing factors include wet and cold environments, wind, age (geriatric/pediatric), medical conditions, substance abuse (alcohol, drugs), and poison. Up to 50% of trauma patients with severe injuries become hypothermic because of exposure, blood loss, shock, and standard procedures (such as administration of cold fluids and clothing removal). Indications of hypothermia include cold skin, shivering, decreased mental status (confusion, memory loss, lethargy, dizziness, mood changes, impaired judgment, difficulty speaking), decreased sensation of touch, decreased motor function (muscle rigidity, stiff posture, muscle/joint stiffness), and bradycardia (slow pulse). Prehospital: Remove the patient from the cold environment, remove any wet clothing, wrap in warm blankets, begin CPR if no pulse is obtained after 30–45 seconds of assessment, and use an AED if it indicates the need to defibrillate.

Frostbite/Freezing

Frostbite is tissue damage from **freezing**, most often affecting the nose, ears, and distal extremities (hands/feet). The affected part feels numb and aches or throbs, becoming hard and insensate as the

- 65 -

tissue freezes, resulting in circulatory impairment, necrosis of tissue, and gangrene. Degrees of frostbite/freezing are as follows:

1. Partial freezing with redness and mild swelling, stinging, burning, and throbbing pain.
2. Full-thickness freezing with increased swelling in 3–4 hours and clear blisters in 6–24 hours; sloughing of skin with eschar formation, numbness, and then aching and throbbing pain.
3. Full-thickness freezing into subdermal tissue with cyanosis, hemorrhagic blisters, skin necrosis, a "wooden" feeling, severe burning, throbbing, and shooting pains.
4. Freezing extends into the subcutaneous tissue (muscles, tendons, and bones) with a mottled appearance, nonblanching cyanosis, and eventually deep black eschar.

Prehospital: Remove the patient from the cold environment, handling him or her with care; remove wet clothing; cover the patient with a blanket; remove jewelry; manually stabilize the affected area; and transport rapidly. Do NOT break blisters, rub or massage the area, apply heat, rewarm if the area may refreeze, allow the patient to walk, or give him or her anything by mouth.

Heat-related illnesses

Condition	Characteristics	Prehospital
Heat stress	Increased temperature causes dehydration. Symptoms may include swelling of the hands and feet, flushing, itching, sunburn, dizziness, muscle cramps, and hyperventilation. The patient's temperature is normal.	Remove the patient from heat and give fluids to rehydrate; give oxygen with a nonrebreather mask.
Heat exhaustion	Dehydration results in sodium depletion. Symptoms may include flu-like symptoms, headache, dizziness, fainting, nausea, vomiting, weakness, muscle cramping, rapid pulse, diaphoresis, and cold clammy skin. The patient's temperature is usually <106°F (41°C), and it may be normal.	Remove the patient from heat; use evaporative cooling techniques such as ice packs to the axilla, groin, and neck; and rehydrate (give one-half glass of fluid every 15 to 20 minutes). Give oxygen as above.
Heat stroke	Two types may progress to multiorgan dysfunction syndrome with liver and kidney failure and death. Exertional: Sudden onset after exertion. The patient's temperature varies because he or she is still sweating. There is diaphoresis, syncope, and loss of consciousness. Nonexertional: Sudden onset after heat exposure. The temperature is usually >106°F (41°C) rectally or >103°F (39.4°C) orally. There can be mild irritability, decorticate posturing, seizures, coma, and tachycardia.	Remove the patient from heat, apply evaporative cooling and ice packs as above, provide airway/ventilation/oxygenation support as needed, and provide rapid transport.

Submersion/drowning

Submersion may cause aspiration (wet drowning) or trigger severe laryngospasm (dry drowning), although some people will be pulled from the water still breathing. **Drowning** is the leading cause of death in children younger than 5, and it is the second leading cause of death in children under 15. Most infant submersions are in bathtubs and result from intentional injury or lack of supervision. Adolescent/Adult submersions are often related to drugs, alcohol, or risk-taking behaviors. Submersion asphyxiation can cause profound damage to multiorgan systems, including the brain, heart, and lungs, from lack of oxygen and aspiration. Hypothermia related to near drowning has some protective effect because blood is shunted to the brain and heart. Indications of submersion include coughing, vomiting, difficulty breathing, and respiratory and cardiac arrest. Prehospital: Initiate CPR if the patient is in arrest, manage the patient's airway/ventilation/oxygen supplementation with 100% oxygen (the patient may need intubation), place the patient in the recovery position if he or she is unconscious or vomiting, provide suction as needed, and provide rapid transport.

Multisystem trauma

Multisystem trauma (common) involves injury to more than one major system. Care includes the following points:

- Ensure the safety of the patient and all rescue personnel, and determine the need for additional resources.
- Consider the mechanism of injury and identify and manage life-threatening conditions.
- Manage the patient's airway/ventilation/oxygen supplementation (high concentration) as well as the necessary spinal immobilization with him or her in a lying/sitting position, and make positioning decisions.
- Control hemorrhage and provide shock therapy and maintain body temperature.
- Splint musculoskeletal injuries.
- Suspect additional injuries.
- Prioritize interventions and continue care en route rather than delaying transport.
- Evaluate the patient's condition by the injuries sustained (bleeding, difficulty breathing, lack of pulse) rather than by the patient's response (screaming, yelling).
- Complete the primary and secondary assessments, and obtain a medical history.
- Platinum ten—the first 10 minutes on the scene in which the patient should be extricated and stabilization efforts should be started.
- Golden hour—the first 60 minutes during which the patient should be stabilized and transported to the receiving facility.
- Notify the receiving facility so resources are prepared.

Special Patient Populations

Premonitory signs of labor

Lightening	As the fetal head engages and moves toward the birth canal, the fundal pressure on the diaphragm lessens, so the mother can breathe more easily, but pressure in the pelvic area increases, causing urinary frequency. The lower abdomen may protrude more than previously. Increased circulatory impairment may cause venous stasis and ankle swelling as well as increased vaginal secretions as the vaginal mucous membranes become congested. Pressure on the nerves may result in leg cramps or pelvic and leg pain.
Braxton Hicks (BH)	BH contractions are short in duration, occur at irregular intervals in the lower abdomen, and do not change the cervix. They are often relieved by activity or mild analgesia. The intensity and frequency of BH contractions often increase immediately prior to the onset of true labor.
Cervical changes	The cervix ripens (softens) to allow for effacement (thinning) and dilation.
Bloody show	A mucous plug from pooled secretions forms at the opening of the cervical canal during pregnancy, and when the cervix begins to efface, this mucous plug is expelled, exposing capillary vessels that bleed. The bloody show typically appears as pink mucus. Bloody show usually occurs within 24 to 48 hours of the onset of labor.
Ruptured membranes	Rupture of the membranes occurs in about 12% of women prior to the onset of labor, which usually then occurs within 24 hours. Before rupture, the membranes typically bulge through the dilating cervix; fluid comes in a gush, although it may come in smaller spurts in some cases. If the membranes rupture before engagement of the fetal head, the umbilical cord may prolapse with the fluid, increasing risk to the fetus, so mothers should always seek medical attention after rupture. If the mother is at term and labor does not start within 24 hours of rupture, labor may be induced.

Stages of labor

First	Latent phase: The cervix begins to dilate; contractions are mild to moderate and occur every 3–30 minutes and are of short duration. Active phase: The cervix is dilated to 4–7 cm; contractions are every 1–5 minutes, lasting 20–40 seconds. Pain is increased. Transitional phase: The cervix is fully dilated (8–10 cm); contractions come every 1.5–2 minutes, lasting 60–90 seconds. There is increased pain, hyperventilation, crying, moaning, vomiting, and rectal pressure.
Second	From fully dilated cervix to delivery with contractions as in the transitional phase. The perineum begins to bulge, and the fetal head crowns as the mother begins to bear down and birth is imminent. Pressure on the rectum and anus may cause stool to be expelled. Birth occurs head first if it is a normal delivery, feet first if it is a breech delivery.
Third	Delivery of the placenta should occur 5–30 minutes after birth. Retained placenta occurs if more than 30 minutes elapse.
Fourth	The period of 1–4 hours after birth, which involves 250–400 mL blood loss, moderate hypotension (low BP), and tachycardia (rapid pulse).

Organs of pregnancy and vaginal bleeding

Organs of pregnancy include the uterus (womb). The placenta is attached to the walls of the uterus; it includes the umbilical cord, which provides blood, nutrients, and oxygen to the fetus. The fetus is inside an amniotic sac, which contains amniotic fluid that cushions the fetus. The opening to the uterus is the cervix, which thins and dilates for delivery. The vagina provides the birth canal. **Vaginal bleeding** during the first trimester of pregnancy may indicate spontaneous abortion, ectopic pregnancy, or infection, although light occasional spotting may be normal. All vaginal bleeding during pregnancy should be assessed by a physician, and a large amount of bleeding may indicate a medical emergency. "Bloody show" near term may indicate that delivery is near. Prehospital: Use standard precautions, and position the patient on her left side. Place a sanitary pad over the vaginal opening and save any soaked pads in a plastic bag so the physician can estimate the blood loss. Manage the patient's airway/ventilation/oxygen supplementation, and provide emotional support.

Delivery of a newborn

If the fetal head is obvious at the vaginal opening (crowning), **delivery** is imminent. Steps to delivery include the following:

- Wash hands and don PPE for standard precautions and obtain an OB kit and supplies.
- Position the patient on her back with hips elevated, knees bent, and legs apart.
- Position one person at the mother's head for support if possible while the other supports the baby's head during delivery.
- Provide oxygen to the mother.
- If the umbilical cord is around the baby's neck, attempt to slip it over the infant's head.
- Make note of the time of delivery.
- Lower the infant's head to facilitate drainage of fluids, and keep the mouth and nose suctioned with a bulb syringe.
- Clamp the cord or cut it if sterile equipment is available.
- Monitor the infant's airway, breathing, and circulation with the baby at the level of the birth canal.
- Monitor delivery of the placenta (afterbirth).
- If mother and infant are stable, allow the infant to nurse.
- Place a sanitary pad over the vaginal opening to contain any bleeding. Observe for hemorrhage.
- Massage the uterus in a circular motion to prevent excessive bleeding.

Initial care of the newborn

Dr. Virginia Apgar developed the **APGAR assessment** in 1952. APGAR stands for **a**ppearance, **p**ulse, **g**rimace, **a**ctivity, and **r**espiration. The APGAR is the first test given to a newborn. It is used as a quick evaluation of a newborn's physical condition to determine if any emergency medical care is needed, and it is administered 1 minute and 5 minutes after birth. The test is administered more than once because the baby's condition may change rapidly. It may be administered for a third time 10 minutes after birth, if needed. The baby is rated on the five subscales, and scores are added together.

A total score of ≥7 is a sign of good health.

Sign	0	1	2
Appearance (skin color)	Cyanotic or pallor over entire body	Normal, except for the extremities	Entire body is normal.
Pulse (heart rate)	Absent	<100 bpm	>100 bpm.
Grimace (reflex irritability)	Unresponsive	Grimace	Infant sneezes, coughs, and recoils.
Activity (muscle tone)	Absent	Flexed limbs	Infant moves freely.
Respiration (breathing rate and effort)	Absent	Bradypnea, dyspnea	Good breathing and crying.

Routine care of the newborn

To **establish an airway**, the infant is placed supine with the head slightly extended in the "sniffing" position. A small neck roll may be placed under the shoulders to maintain this position in a very small premature infant. Once the proper position is established, the mouth and nose are suctioned (suction the mouth first to prevent reflex inspiration of secretions when the nose is suctioned) with a bulb syringe or catheter if necessary. The infant's head can be turned momentarily to the side to allow secretions to pool in the cheek where they can be more easily suctioned and removed to establish the airway. **Stimulating** the newborn is often all that is needed to initiate spontaneous respirations. This tactile stimulation can be accomplished by gently rubbing the back or trunk of the infant. Another technique that is used to provide stimulation is flicking or rubbing the soles of the feet. Slapping neonates as stimulation is no longer practiced and should NOT be used. The infant should be given a **rapid assessment** within seconds of birth to determine if he or she is at term, if the amniotic fluid is clear, if there is muscle tone, and if there are respirations or crying. If any of these conditions are not met, then further resuscitation is needed. The basic steps to care include the following:

- Warming the infant after drying.
- Positioning the infant and clearing the airway if necessary.
- Stimulating and repositioning the infant.

The child should be evaluated throughout the initial procedures as follows:

- Respirations: The rate and character of the respirations should be noted as well as an observation of chest wall movement.
- Heart rate: Should be >100 bpm, assessed with a stethoscope or at the base of the umbilical cord.

Infants have poor temperature regulation ability, particularly preterm infants, who lack brown fat, which is one of the body's tools to regulate body temperature, so **providing warmth** is critical as a component of resuscitation. An infant who is just seconds old and wet will need aggressive measures to keep him or her warm while any resuscitation efforts are being initiated. Infants lose heat through their heads, so one of the first steps should be to place a hat on the head or cover the head in some way. The infant should be vigorously dried with warmed blankets. Often, this stimulation—drying and warming—is all that is needed to establish a regular respiration pattern in the neonate. Preterm infants weighing <1500 grams should be placed in a plastic bag (made specifically for this purpose), if available, up to the height of the shoulders to prevent cold shock. A term infant with no apparent distress can be placed on the mother's chest and covered with a warm blanket.

Pediatric assessment

Pediatric assessment should include the following:

- Pediatric assessment triangle:
  - o Appearance (abnormal tone, decreased interactivity, decreased consolability, abnormal look/gaze, and abnormal speech or cry).
  - o Work of breathing (abnormal sounds [wheezing, stridor], position, retractions [sternum], flaring [nostrils], and apnea/gasping).
  - o Circulation (pallor, mottling, and cyanosis).
- Assess airway, breathing, and circulation (heart rate/pulse): Place in the shock position and provide a warming blanket for signs of shock.
- Ventilation/oxygenation: Administer oxygen and assist with ventilation if it is abnormal.
- Determine the patient's level of consciousness: Use the alert, voice, pain, unresponsive (AVPU) assessment. Note movement of the extremities and whether pupils are normal, dilated, constricted, reactive, or fixed.
- Prevent hypothermia: Cover with a warming blanket, cover the head, and avoid unnecessary exposure of the skin.
- Obtain the medical history from the caregiver/parent: Include the type and duration of symptoms, fever, level of activity, recent foods/fluids, medications, medication allergies, past or chronic illnesses, and events leading to the current problem.
- Head-to-toe physical examination: Note any bruising, swelling, drainage, loose teeth, unusual odors, bleeding, rashes, deformities, and pain on movement.

Pediatric seizures

Febrile seizure is a generalized seizure associated with fever (usually >38.8°C [101.8°F]) from any type of infection (upper respiratory, urinary tract) but without intracranial infection or other cause, occurring between 6 months and 5 years of age. Seizures usually last <15 minutes and are without subsequent neurological deficit. Prehospital: Provide fever control (acetaminophen OR ibuprofen) and a tepid-water bath.

Other types of seizures may result from pathology, such as meningitis, cerebral edema, brain trauma, or brain tumors, but most seizures in children >3 are related to idiopathic epilepsy, which predisposes the child to recurrent seizures, usually of the same type. Seizures are characterized as focal (localized), focal with rapid generalization (spreading), and generalized (widespread). In most children, seizures become generalized with loss of consciousness. Seizure disorders with onset younger than 4 years old usually cause more neurological damage than those at older than 4 years. Prehospital: Place the patient on the floor or a safe surface, loosen clothes, and protect from injury during seizure. Afterwards, place the patient in the recovery position, monitor airway/ventilation, and provide oxygenation (the patient may need assisted ventilation if he or she is cyanotic) and suction if needed.

Apparent life-threatening events (ALTEs) and sudden infant death syndrome (SIDS)

Infants with an **apparent life-threatening event (ALTE)** are those who are lifeless and without respirations but are successfully resuscitated or begin breathing spontaneously. With **sudden infant death syndrome (SIDS),** which is almost always related to respiratory arrest, the child

- 71 -

cannot be resuscitated. There are numerous proposed causes for ALTE and SIDS, so a careful history, including familial history of SIDS, and physical examination or postmortem examination can provide important information, such as indications of child abuse or metabolic/infectious disorders. Prehospital: Continue resuscitative efforts (airway/ventilation/oxygenation, compressions as indicated) and stabilize the infant if possible. The child with ALTE should be hospitalized for observation, further studies, and apnea monitoring because these children are at an increased risk for SIDS. For SIDS patients, the paramedic should provide support and information to the family. The protocol for reporting SIDS varies by state, but it usually involves notifying the coroner's office.

Assessing the patient's level of consciousness

The AVPU is a quick assessment done to determine the patient's level of consciousness. This may be one of the first assessments done when initially attending to a patient.

Alert, voice, pain, unresponsive (AVPU)			
A	Alert and awake; aware of person, place, time, and condition. Follows commands. Pediatric: Active and responds to external stimuli and to the caregiver.	Yes	No
V	Responds to verbal stimuli, but the eyes do not open spontaneously. Pediatric: Responds only when the caregiver calls the child's name.	Yes	No
P	Responds to painful stimuli, such as pinching the skin/earlobe, but not to verbal stimuli. Pediatric: Responds only to painful stimuli, such as pinching the nailbed.	Yes	No
U	Unresponsive—does not respond to painful or verbal stimuli. Pediatric: Unresponsive.	Yes	No

Geriatric considerations

Geriatric patients may have the following considerations:

- Decreased sensory input (hearing, vision, touch, pain); impaired depth perception and night vision; and decreased ability to differentiate colors.
- Hypertension, increasing the risk of heart attack and stroke.
- Decreased breathing capacity and decreased cough, increasing the risk of infection.
- Difficulty chewing and swallowing; digestive problems; and reflux when lying flat, increasing the risk of aspiration.
- Short-term memory deficit and slower reflexes.
- Decreased bone density, increasing the risk of breaks; loss of muscle tone.
- Increased risk of infection and less obvious symptoms of infection.
- Arthritis in the neck, interfering with airway assessment.
- Dentures that can obstruct the airway (leave them in place if possible during ventilation).
- Skin that is fragile and tears easily.
- Irregular pulse from underlying heart problems.
- Dementia (incidence increases with age), making history taking and treatment difficult.
- Atypical symptoms for illnesses, even if severely ill.
- Multiple comorbidities and multiple medications.
- Shock with blood pressure (BP) greater than 100.

Elder abuse

Physical	Various types of assault related to hitting, kicking, pulling hair, shoving, and pushing. Patients may be forcibly confined, forced into seclusion, and/or force-fed to the point that they choke on food.
Psychological	Caregivers may threaten to hit the patient, brandish a weapon, and/or tell the person to commit suicide. Ongoing intimidation may make the patient terrified and anxious. Sometimes, caregivers threaten to injure pets or family members, increasing the patient's fear.
Sexual	Types of sexual abuse include the following: Physical: Fondling, kissing, and rape. Emotional: Exhibitionism. Verbal: Sexual harassment, using obscene language, and threatening.
Financial	Financial abuse includes the following: Outright stealing of property or persuading patients to give away possessions. Forcing patients to sign away property. Emptying bank and savings accounts and using stolen credit cards. Convincing the person to invest money in fraudulent schemes. Taking money for home renovations that are not done.

Child abuse

Children rarely admit to **abuse** (physical, sexual, or emotional) and often attempt to protect the abusing parent. Therefore, suspicion of abuse depends on other indicators such as the following:

- **Behavioral:** The child may be overly compliant or fearful with obvious changes in demeanor when a parent/caregiver is present. Some children act out with aggression toward other children or animals. Children may become depressed or suicidal or present with sleeping or eating disorders. Behaviors may become increasingly self-destructive as the child ages, including inappropriate sexualized behavior.
- **Physical/Sexual:** The type, location, and extent of injuries can raise the suspicion of abuse. Head and facial injuries and bruising are common, as are bite or burn marks and spiral fractures. There may be handprints or grab marks and unusual bruising, such as across the buttocks. Any bruising, swelling, or tearing of the genital area and the identification of sexually transmitted diseases are also causes for concern.

Suspected abuse must be reported to the appropriate authorities, according to protocol, with careful documentation of findings and statements by the child or caregivers.

Neglect and lack of supervised care

Children and older or impaired adults may suffer from profound **neglect or a lack of supervision** that places them at risk. Indicators include the following:

- Appearing dirty and unkempt, sometimes with infestations of lice, and wearing ill-fitting, torn clothing and shoes.
- Being tired and sleepy during the daytime.
- Having excessive medical or dental problems, such as extensive dental caries.
- Missing doctor appointments and not receiving proper immunizations.
- Being underweight for their current stage of development.
- Lacking assistive devices or misplaced hearing aids/eyeglasses.

- Left in soiled or urine-/feces-soiled clothing.
- Clothing is inadequate (such as lack of a coat/sweater during winter or dirty, torn, ill-fitting clothes).

Neglect can be difficult to assess, especially if the EMR is serving a homeless or very disadvantaged population. Home visits may be needed to ascertain if there is adequate food, clothing, or supervision, and this is beyond the scope of care provided by the EMR. Thus, suspicions should be reported to the appropriate authorities who can arrange a follow-up assessment of the home environment.

Injuries consistent with domestic violence/abuse

Characteristic injuries	Ruptured eardrum. Rectal/genital injury—burns, bites, trauma. Scrapes and bruises about the neck, face, head, trunk, arms. Cuts, bruises, and fractures of the face.
Patterns of injuries	"Bathing suit" pattern—injuries on parts of body that are usually covered with clothing because the perpetrator wants to hide the evidence of abuse. Head and neck injuries (50%).
Abusive injuries (rarely attributable to accidents)	Bites, bruises, rope and cigarette burns, and welts in the outline of weapons (belt marks). Bilateral injuries of the arms/legs.
Defensive injuries	Back-of-the-body injury from being attacked while crouched on the floor facedown. Located on the soles of the feet from kicking at a perpetrator. Located on the ulnar aspect of the hands or palm from blocking blows.

EMS Operations

Apparatus and equipment readiness

The EMR should ensure that the ambulance is ready for use and that the tires are properly inflated, the gas tank is full, warning devices are working, and engine fluid levels are appropriate. All necessary safety equipment, such as PPE (masks, gowns, gloves, and goggles or face guards) and safety devices (safety vests, road flares, and signs) as well as seat belts and harnesses, should be available and in proper working condition. All equipment in the cab, the compartments, and the rear of the ambulance should be in the proper place, labeled, and secured to prevent shifting during transportation. High-risk situations include going through intersections, inclement weather (especially with poor visibility), careless drivers, highway access, unpaved roads, and driver distractions (conversation, eating, drinking, mobile devices, music, GPS devices, and fatigue). During transportation, all personnel as well as patients should be properly secured with safety equipment.

Scene-of-incident safety considerations

The EMR must do a 360° **assessment of the scene** of incident on arrival and determine safety considerations. The EMR should make note of any gunshots heard, downed power lines, buildings in a state of collapse, leaking fuels/fluids, fire, smoke, broken glass, and other hazards. The EMR may need to wait until the site is safe to proceed. The EMR should assess the mechanism of injury (accidents) and the need for appropriate PPE (gloves, gown, mask, face guard) and must keep the patient informed of all actions and prevent harm or further injury. The ambulance should be parked off of the roadway if possible or parked at a 45° angle (front wheels out) to shield the work area, making sure not to block access for other emergency vehicles. Parking uphill is safer than downhill and upwind rather than downwind. If flares are used to warn other drivers, they should extend at least 300 feet from a collision. Yellow warning lights at the scene are the safest, but excessive lighting may blind other drivers at night.

Transferring a patient from the scene to an ambulance

Different types of **stretchers** and **transfer equipment** may be used for prehospital transfer, including the following:

- Wheeled: Stretcher that can be lowered and raised with a wheeled base allowing it to slide into the ambulance.
- Scoop: Two- to four-piece stretcher that can be connected and placed under a patient.
- Transfer sheet: A heavy plastic sheet can be used with patients up to 800 lb to facilitate transfer.
- Flexible stretcher: Lightweight flexible (plastic, rubberized canvas) stretcher with webbing handles on both sides. Can be used to transfer patients around corners and up and down stairs where a wheeled stretcher cannot be used.
- Stair chair: Safety chair that can be used to transfer patients in tight spaces and up and down stairs.
- Lightweight stretcher: Folding stretcher made of lightweight materials.
- Basket stretcher (Stokes basket): Used primarily for rescues in the wilderness or from cliffs.

Patient positioning should be according to the possible or probable injury, with safety restraints always securing the patient to the gurney and the gurney to the vehicle.

- Left-side-lying: Pregnant patients should be placed in this position to increase circulation to the placenta, and unconscious patients should be placed in this position to prevent aspiration and choking if there is no indication of a spinal injury.
- Supine (flat on the back): Patient has a suspected pelvic fracture or neck injury (also requires a cervical collar).
- Supine (feet elevated above the heart): This is the position for patients in shock to increase circulation to the heart and brain as the BP falls.
- Trendelenburg (the entire stretcher is tilted so that the head is below the feet): Position for patients with a suspected spinal cord injury.
- Semi-Fowler's (30- to 45-degree position): For patients with chest pain, stroke, and/or shortness of breath and no indication of a spinal cord injury.
- Fowler's (upright, 90-degree position): For patients with severe shortness of breath.

Environmental risk factors

When assessing a patient, it's important to consider that **environmental factors** may place the patient at an increased risk for harm or may be a factor in disease. There are a number of different types of environmental factors to consider.

Factors	Examples	Effects
Toxic chemicals	Lead, arsenic, muriatic acid, sulfuric acid, ammonia, lime	May result in poisoning (lead, arsenic) or burns (acids, ammonia, lime) through direct exposure or inhalation
Physical objects	Guns, cars, knives, equipment	Accidents, gunshot wounds, stabbings, various injuries (blunt and penetrating)
Biological organisms	Bacteria, fungi, viruses	Infections
Temperature variations	Heat, cold	Burns, dehydration, heat stroke, hyperthermia, hypothermia, frostbite
Ambient noise	Sirens, loud music, traffic noise, work-related noise	Hearing loss/deafness, increased anxiety
Psychosocial	Increased stress	Anxiety, hypertension, suicidal ideation

Rescues in confined spaces

A **confined space** is one in which access is limited and the space is surrounded by walls or structures that are not suitable for habitation. A confined space may occur in a building (such as with a collapse), a silo, a motor vehicle (such as a large vehicle involved in a crash), a cistern or septic tank, or a well. A confined space may pose a risk to the patient and the EMR because of difficulty moving about and accessing the patient as well as decreased ventilation that may result in the buildup of toxic gases and/or a lack of oxygen. Before entering a confined space, the EMR should test the atmosphere and use the correct breathing equipment. This is especially important if the patient is nonresponsive, which is often an indication of poor air quality. The EMR should also carefully assess his or her ability to access the patient and the best means of doing so.

Driving safety

The **ambulance driver** should stop briefly or slow significantly at intersections because other drivers may not hear or may ignore sirens. The driver should keep the brake covered with the left foot for fast braking and avoid excessive speeds because of the increased risk of accidents, especially on curves. The speed should be adjusted for road and weather conditions and should not be influenced by use of the siren (siren syndrome). Snow and ice should be cleared from the ambulance before driving it. At least one vehicle length should separate the ambulance from other vehicles for every 10 mph of speed. A spotter should always be used when backing up the ambulance because of poor visibility. All personnel in the ambulance should be seated and secured with seat belts or safety harnesses before the ambulance moves. Studies have shown that CPR is most effective if done from a sitting position in an ambulance rather than standing, despite common practice. Patients and gurneys should also be secured.

Lights and sirens

Lights and sirens should be used together, and they are indicated when going to a scene and when transporting a patient in a serious emergent situation. There are four types of warning lights used on emergency vehicles such as ambulances: rotating lights (resulting in a flashing sensation), fixed flashes (usually red or blue), strobe lights, and LED lights. Red (the most common) and blue lights are generally used to indicate emergency vehicles and can be used to obtain the right-of-way or to block the right-of-way. These colors may be interchangeable, although in some states the color blue is restricted to law enforcement vehicles. Amber lights are warning lights and can be used by all vehicles, but they do not require others to stop. Some emergency vehicle lights change to amber when the vehicle is parked. White warning lights cannot be used on the rear of an emergency vehicle. Green lights are sometimes used to indicate a mobile incident command post, but in some states, green lights may also indicate private security vehicles or volunteer firefighters.

Incident management

FEMA IS-700.A outlines the **National Incident Management System (NIMS)**, which, under the direction of the Federal Emergency Management Agency (FEMA), an agency of the U.S. Department of Homeland Security, provides the foundation for collaboration among different governmental and nongovernmental agencies, jurisdictions, and specialties/disciplines in handling large-scale incidents that threaten life, property, and/or the environment. Components of FEMA IS-700.A include the following:

- Preparedness: Focuses on planning, procedures and protocols, training and exercises, personnel qualifications/certification, and equipment certification, and it includes the National Response Framework, which ensures that local jurisdictions retain control but use a unified approach and establishes protocols.
- Communications and information management: Systems must be interoperable, reliable, portable, scalable, resilient, and redundant.
- Resource management: Includes personnel, equipment, supplies, and facilities, which must be inventoried and categorized using a standardized approach.
- Command and management: Includes the Incident Command System (this standardized approach outlines the responsibilities of the incident commander, area command, command staff, and general staff), multiagency coordination systems, and public information.
- Management and maintenance: The National Integration Center (NIC) is responsible for NIMS management.

- Flexibility: Components are scalable and adaptable to all types of incidents.
- Standardization: The NIC develops standards.

ICS-100.B, the **Incident Command System** course, meets NIMS requirements for operational personnel and outlines a standardized approach to incident management. ICS is used for any type of major event, planned or otherwise, and large- or small-scale incidents, including natural (disasters), technological (hazmat release), and human-caused (civil disturbance) hazards. ICS outlines the chain of command (the incident commander in control and orders going through supervisors). Every incident requires an incident action plan, resource management, and processes for reimbursement. The incident commander establishes an incident command post and staging areas (gathering places) as well a base (coordination area for logistic and administrative functions), camps (for sleeping, eating, and sanitary services), helibases, and helispots. Primary features of ICS include common terminology, establishment/transfer of command, chain of command/unity of command, management of objects, incident action planning, modular organization, manageable span of control, comprehensive resource management, incident facilities and locations, integrated communications, information and intelligence management, accountability, and dispatch/deployment.

Each organization must establish the **chain of command** for its incident command system. Although these may vary somewhat, an incident commander is ultimately in charge with individuals being assigned as incident managers in different areas, such as triage, treatment, transport, security, and liaison. **Unity of command** means that each incident commander should have control over personnel assigned to his or her area and each individual within the chain of command should have a clear understanding of whom to report to at the scene so that communication is efficient and timely. **Unified command** means that when multiple agencies are involved from multiple jurisdictions, the chain of command that has been established is recognized and respected even though each agency retains its own authority and accountability and is responsible for carrying out its own duties. A unified command system prevents duplication of effort as well as neglect of important functions.

The purpose of the **incident action plan** is to outline control objectives, resources, and strategies for dealing with an incident. Incident action plans should be updated frequently. Incident action plans may be designed for various types of incidents (terrorist attack, disease outbreak, hurricane) and modified as needed and should include the following:

- Goals and objectives, including expected outcomes.
- Strategies and tactics for responding and accomplishing the goals and objectives.
- An outline of the chain of command for the incident command system, including the span of control (the number of people reporting to an individual).
- Tasks assigned to each level in the chain of command.
- Safety/Health plan for responders to prevent injury/illness and to treat as needed.
- Communications plan outlining how information will be exchanged, including alternative methods of command if, for example, cell phone towers are out of commission.
- Logistics plan regarding the acquisition and use of resources, such as supplies, personnel, and equipment.
- Maps and demographic information.

When a multiple-casualty or mass-casualty event occurs, the first lead emergency medical responder on the scene generally assumes the role of **incident commander** and carries out a rapid assessment of the scene and begins to call for additional resources as indicated while another medical responder begins triage. The incident commander should begin to establish a command center in an area that is safe and out of the way of emergency vehicles while awaiting assistance. This first incident commander will relinquish the role when the staffed and/or assigned incident commander arrives to take command and should then report to the person who is assuming the role of staging officer. The incident commander's duties include establishing command, assessing needs, developing a plan, coordinating all activities, delegating responsibilities, ensuring the safety of all personnel and patients, liaising with other agencies, and communicating information.

Multiple-casualty incidents

Primary triage is a rapid method (30 to 60 seconds) of prioritizing patients based on the severity of their condition, and it is carried out at the scene of multiple-casualty incidents. All patients are triaged and tagged according to the following international color-coding priority (P) guidelines on the foot or wrist (not on the clothing):

- P1—Red: Immediate care is needed for urgent systemic life-threatening conditions, such as airway/breathing problems, severe bleeding, severe burns (especially with breathing problems), decreased mental status, shock, and severe medical problems, or a Glasgow Coma Scale score of ≤13.
- P2—Yellow: Delayed care and able to wait 45–60 minutes for treatment. Conditions include burns (without breathing problems), multiple bone/joint injuries, back and/or spinal cord injuries (unless the patient is in respiratory distress).
- P3—Green: Hold, able to wait hours for treatment of minor injuries.
- P4—Black: Deceased.

Resource management involves identifying a triage officer who remains at the scene during the event and identifying the need for additional personnel and equipment and providing those to the patients with the highest priority.

During a mass-casualty incident, triage is done quickly, and patients may be scattered over a wide area with many patients being red-tagged for emergency care. Patients coded black are left in place, but those with other-color tags should be moved and segregated in separate sections of a holding area to await treatment and/or transport. The patients should be **retriaged** as they are moved into the holding area to determine if the tagging color is still appropriate. Additionally, **secondary triage** may be carried out in the separate sections, especially if some must be airlifted, to determine which of the patients have the best chance of survival and should receive priority for transfer and treatment. Secondary triage may also help to determine which trauma center (based on location or level of care) or hospital is most appropriate for the patient considering the patient's condition, transport time, and the surge capacity of the healthcare institutions.

Centers for Disease Control and Prevention guidelines for field triage of injured patients

The **CDC's guidelines for field triage** of injured patients is a four-step algorithm that is used to identify the most seriously ill patients and transport them to an appropriate treatment center.

Step	Assess	Findings requiring priority treatment	Plan
1	Vital signs/Level of consciousness	Glasgow Coma Scale score of ≤13, systolic BP <90 mm Hg, respiratory rate <10 or >29 per minute (<20 in an infant <1 year), or need of ventilatory support.	Highest level trauma center
2	Anatomy of injury	Penetrating injuries, flail chest, two or more long-bone fractures, crushed/mangled/pulseless extremity, amputations, pelvic fractures, open/depressed skull fracture, or paralysis.	Highest level trauma center
3	Mechanism of injury/High-energy impact	Falls—adults >20 feet and children >10 feet or 2–3 times their height. High-risk auto crash with intrusions, partial or complete ejection, or there is a death in the same passenger compartment. Auto vs. pedestrian/bicycle with victim thrown, run over, or sustaining a significant impact. Motorcycle crash >20 mph.	Trauma center
4	Special patient/system considerations	Older adults, children, pregnancy >30 weeks, burns, patients on anticoagulants or with bleeding disorders (based on the EMR's best judgment).	Trauma center/Hospital

START method of triage

With the **START method of triage**, the paramedic starts triage with the first victim encountered, tags the patient, and then moves to the next patient, assessing in order: (1) respirations, (2) perfusion, and (3) mental status (RPM) and using the standard red-yellow-green-black color-coding system. Walking wounded are tagged as green.

Respirations	Present.	Red tag if >30. Continue to perfusion assessment if <30.
	Not present—position the airway.	Red tag if respirations recur or black tag (death) if none.
Perfusion	Radial pulse absent or capillary refill of greater than 2 seconds.	Control bleeding and red tag.
	Radial pulse present and capillary refill time of less than 2 seconds.	Continue to mental status assessment.
Mental status	Cannot follow simple directions.	Red tag.
	Can follow simple directions.	Yellow tag.

JumpSTART method of triage for pediatric patients

JumpSTART is a pediatric triage method developed only for use in multiple-casualty incidents.

Able to walk	No	Continue to breathing assessment.
	Yes	Green tag. Carry out secondary triage.
Breathing	No	Step 1: Position upper airway and red tag if breathing. Step 2: Give five rescue breaths and red tag if breathing. Black tag if breathing does not recur.
	Yes	Respiratory rate <15 or >45, red tag. Respiratory rate 15 to 45, continue to pulse assessment.
Palpable pulse	No	Red tag.
	Yes	Continue to AVPU assessment.
Alert, voice, pain, unresponsive (AVPU) assessment	Inappropriate pain, posturing, or unresponsive	Red tag.
	A, V, or P is appropriate	Yellow tag.

Multiple-casualty incidents

Critical incident stress management (CISM) is a procedure to help people cope with stressful events, such as disasters, in order to reduce the incidence of post-traumatic stress syndrome (PTSS).

- Defusing sessions usually occur very early, sometimes during or immediately after a stressful event, and they are used to educate personnel who are actively involved about what to expect over the next few days and to provide guidance in handling their feelings and stress levels.
- Debriefing sessions usually follow in one to three days and may be repeated periodically as needed. These sessions may include people who were directly involved as well as those who were indirectly involved. People are encouraged to express their emotions about the event. Critiquing the event or attempting to place blame is not productive as part of the CISM process.
- Follow-up is done at the end of the process, usually after about week, but this time frame can vary.

Air medical transport

Air medical transport is indicated when the patient is in need of a high level of care that may be available on an aircraft but not an ambulance, when the patient's condition and need for treatment are time critical, when the patient is located in a remote area where access by ambulance is difficult or would be delayed (helicopter), or when local medical services have exceeded their capacity. Helipads are often available at large hospitals, so the patient can be treated immediately after arrival. Some disadvantages include inclement weather (which may interfere with flight plans) as well as altitude and airspeed limitations. Depending on the aircraft, the cabin size may be inadequate for the patient, personnel, and equipment. Difficult terrain, such as forested or hilly areas may not provide an adequate landing site. Cost is the biggest difference between ground and air transport with air transport often costing tens of thousands of dollars with only part, or in some cases none, of the costs being covered by insurance.

Helicopters have the advantage over fixed-wing aircraft of being able to load a patient at or near the scene rather than having to transport the patient by ambulance to an airport. A paved surface is not necessary for a helicopter landing site, but level grassy or paved sites are preferred, ideally with 100 × 100 feet of clear space, but a minimum area of 60 × 60 feet may be used. Additionally, the area should be free of debris that may be disrupted by the rotor blades and should be clear of structures that may interfere with the aircraft, such as power poles, tall trees, power lines, cables, and antennas. A rotor aircraft does not require that people approach in a crouching position, but people should avoid holding anything over their heads and should generally approach from the front of the aircraft and avoid the rear of the aircraft and the rear rotors.

The pilot in command (PIC) of rotorcraft and fixed-wing aircraft is responsible for the **safety** of the aircraft, crew, emergency medical personnel, and the patient. As with all takeoffs and landings, medical staff and crew must be seated and secured by seat belts. Helmets should be in place and secure. Patients who are violent, confused, or combative should be physically restrained for transport and may also require chemical restraints to ensure their own personal safety as well as the safety of the medical and flight crew. Patients should be offloaded ONLY when a crew member signals the receiving medical personnel to approach the aircraft. With high-altitude fixed-wing air transports, cabins are pressurized but only to the equivalent of 6000–8000 feet, not to sea level. Rotorcraft are usually used to transfer a patient from the scene of an incident to a primary care facility or from the primary care facility to another type of facility, whereas a fixed-wing aircraft is usually used from one facility to another over longer distances.

Communication issues associated with air medical services

A **communication specialist** should coordinate all air medical services, including communications within an agency and between agencies regarding all aspects of transport. The communication specialist should have radio communication skills and knowledge of medical terminology, including knowledge of how to obtain information about a patient, navigation, map usage, customer service, weather, aircraft emergencies, as well as FAA and Federal Communications Commission (FCC) regulations that relate to air medical transport. The communication specialist should be familiar with radio frequencies used by EMS. The dispatcher determines whether an aircraft should take off. The communication center may be located in a medical facility, airport, or other space, but it should be free of distractions and have emergency backup electrical power. All air medical transport team members should have knowledge of the radio communication system. Some systems include radio or radio-phone communication, and some systems require the team members to carry pagers, such as two-way satellite pagers. All incoming and outgoing communication should be recorded.

State and federal regulations regarding air medical services

State **statutes** require that aircraft used for air ambulance service must be licensed to provide that service, and the service must ensure that all required medical equipment is available. Although statutes may vary slightly from one state to another, most require that the service be able to provide basic and advanced life support and should provide patients with a description of services and costs. Additionally, the aircraft and crew must comply with Federal Aviation Administration (FAA) regulations and carry insurance to cover injuries that may occur in transport. The FAA carries out periodic inspections of aircraft and issues resource documents regarding safety and operations. Federal regulations establish weather guidelines for safe flying. The U.S. Department of Transportation provides guidelines regarding standards of care. The Commission on Accreditation of Medical Transport Systems establishes voluntary accreditation standards, but air medical services associated with hospitals must meet hospital accreditation standards, typically those of the Joint Commission.

Safe extrication from a motor vehicle (car, truck)

Scene management at the site of an accident that requires a vehicle extrication incudes initial evaluation of any hazards at the site (360° evaluation), such as oncoming traffic, fallen wires, spilled fuel, and fire/explosion risk or presence. The scene must be secured (45° parking, police security, flares, and cones), and the EMR should don protective equipment as necessary and access the patient to provide life-saving care. The patient must be disentangled from the motor vehicle as much as can be done safely. The patient is prepared for extrication (such as by applying pressure to bleeding sites and placing a cervical collar), removed from the vehicle, and then prepared for ground or air transport and provided emergent treatment. For extrications in difficult terrain, assess the following:

- Terrain: Forests, desert, cliff, water, snow.
- Obstacles: Trees, rocks, light, unavailability of landing sites.
- Methods to be used: Helicopter extrication, overland carry, type of extrication.
- Alternative solutions: Abort; contact search and rescue.
- Safety issues: Review all safety concerns.

For **vehicle extrication,** the vehicle must be stabilized before the EMS personnel attempt to enter the vehicle or administer aid to the patient, especially if the vehicle may slide or is on its side and the personnel must access the vehicle from the top because the vehicle may shift and further endanger the patient as well as EMS personnel. EMS personnel can access the vehicle through a window (breaking it if necessary) or a door if one is operable (the patient may be able to assist in opening a window or door). EMS personnel should carry an airway (in case the patient requires ventilation), dressings (to apply pressure if the patient is bleeding), and a rigid cervical collar (to protect against spinal injury or further spinal damage) and should do rapid triage on access to the patient. Oxygen is usually not administered until after the patient is extracted because of the danger of fire, especially if the patient is saturated with fuel, and CPR is not done until the patient is in the supine position on a solid surface. If patients are apneic and pulseless, they must be removed as quickly as possible even with only manual protection of the spine being provided.

For **vehicle extrication**, once EMS personnel have gained access to the motor vehicle, they should unlock its doors if possible to allow others to more easily gain access. EMS personnel should ensure that the engine is turned off, the parking brake is set, and the transmission is set to park. If possible, an emergency response person should disconnect the battery to decrease the risk of fire and explosion. If the patient can be removed, a short backboard should be applied before moving the patient. If the patient is wedged between the seat and the steering wheel, the seat may be slid back manually while rescuers support the patient. If the seat has become dislodged from the track, then the patient should be completely immobilized because this type of mechanical damage can result in severe physical injury. If the patient's legs are trapped, lifting the steering wheel away may also lift the dashboard and help to release the patient.

If a patient must be **cut from a vehicle** (such as when the vehicle is on its side and access must be through a U-shaped flap in the roof), he or she should be warned of the noise and should be covered with a safety blanket (heavy aluminized). In some accidents, **air bags** may not deploy, but movement of the patient or vehicle may cause them to deploy, resulting in danger to the patient and EMS personnel. If the air bags have not deployed, then the battery cables should be disconnected or cut (negative side first) to prevent deployment and personnel should avoid being in front of the path of deployment. EMS personnel should check for side air bags as well as front. The air bags should be deactivated before the steering column is moved (keeping in mind that deactivation can take up to 30 minutes), and care should be taken to avoid cutting or drilling into an air bag.

Since the 1990s, vehicles have been equipped with **seat belt pretensioners** on three-point (shoulder harness) systems in the front and often also in the back. The purpose of seat belt pretensioners is to tighten any slack in the belts in an accident, pulling the person back into the seat and in the proper position for deployment of the air bag. Evidence of pretensioners is not always visible, although an accordion sleeve near the buckle end may be an indication. This sleeve compresses if the pretensioner fires. Although an undeployed pretensioner poses less threat to EMS personnel than an undeployed air bag, it can increase the risk of injury to the patient or EMS personnel, so the seat belt should be disconnected or cut immediately on access to the patient. If the patient was not wearing the seat belt on impact and the pretensioner fired, the seat belt will be tightly vertical along pillar B. If the seat belt pretensioner fired while being worn, it will be extended and will not be retractable.

Although large and heavy pieces of equipment, such as hydraulic rescue tools (including the Jaws of Life, cutters, spreaders, truck jacks, and rams), pneumatic tools, and come-along tools, are often used in vehicle extrication, a tool kit with **simple hand tools** should also be readily available. They may also be needed to access and safely remove a patient from a vehicle. Tools that may be needed for disassembly include adjustable wrenches, screwdrivers (flat and Phillips), flashlight, penlight, medical scissors, headlamp, pliers, bolt cutters, hammers, axes, crowbars, rescue knives (specially designed to cut through seat belts and clothing), and tin snips. Combination rescue tools are available that can be used for a variety of purposes, such as shutting off gas valves, prying open windows, and cutting through battery cables. Tool belt pouches are available to hold small tools that may be needed during an extrication.

Cribbing and chocking are used to raise a vehicle and prevent it from rolling, such as when a patient is caught beneath a vehicle. Cribbing consists of 2×4 blocks and wedges and 4×4 blocks and wedges that are used to create crib boxes to hold an air bag. Cribs are usually made of Douglas fir or southern yellow pine, which can hold 500 psi and crushes slowly. The cribbing is stacked with a 4-inch overhang (to allow for compression), and it should not exceed 48 inches in height. The crib box is put in place with the air bag on top. Chocks are large stepped wedges that are placed in front of or behind wheels to keep them from rolling when the air bag is inflated. As the air bag is slowly inflated, capture cribbing stacks are placed on both sides behind it to hold the vehicle when the air bag is deflated. Once the vehicle is elevated and secured, the air bag is deflated and the crib box is removed to allow room for extrication of the patient.

Some vehicles are powered by **alternative fuels**, such as compressed natural gas (CNG) or liquefied natural gas (LNG), so EMS personnel should look for CNG/LNG logos, often on the right rear or near the refueling port or the right rear of the cab (semitruck). A "natural gas vehicle" warning may be located near the bottom of the rear doors. CNG tanks may be located behind cabs in semitractors, and some may have additional saddle tanks. The power should be turned off, and the 12-volt battery positive and negative cables should be cut. The emergency shut-off valve should be located and turned off, although each tank can also be turned off manually. Electric vehicles pose the risk of stranded energy. Batteries should always be considered energized with a potential for high-voltage injury. Damaged lithium ion batteries that are leaking or sparking are at risk for thermal runaway (fire). The car battery should be shut down immediately. If the battery is damaged, the vehicle must be relocated at least 50 feet from any combustible material.

Bus extrication

Before accessing patients involved in a **bus crash,** the bus must be stabilized, especially if it is on its side or if it is upside down. If the engine is still running, a stop button is often located on the left side of the front panel. Access to the bus may be through the front door if possible. Access may also be through the front windshield (which can be removed through removal of the rubber locking strip that surrounds the window), side windows, the emergency exit door or window, the bathroom window, or an opening cut into the top of the vehicle. Removal of injured patients (usually on stretchers) from inside the vehicle often requires rapid triage and the assistance of multiple EMS personnel. If the vehicle remains upright but patients are completely or partially beneath the vehicle, they should be removed quickly because they may be crushed if the air suspension system deflates.

Aircraft extrication

Communication is essential if EMS personnel are responding to an **aircraft crash site** because they need to know when the crash occurred, the type and size of the aircraft, the number of passengers and crew, reports of fire or explosion, and whether the aircraft is private, commercial, or military, as well as the status (fire, collapse) of any structure(s) that the aircraft may have impacted. For a small plane with the cabin still reasonably intact, extrication may be similar to a motor vehicle, but severe crashes in which the cabin is destroyed and large airplane crashes pose significantly different problems because passengers may have been thrown about inside or outside of the aircraft and seats and belongings and body parts may block access. Victims may lie in the roadway, so emergency vehicles must proceed with caution. Fire and explosions may be a severe risk, and rescuers may need to wait for fire suppression. Triage may begin outside of the aircraft while the aircraft (or the remains of the aircraft) is secured.

Extrication considerations

Part of the stabilization of the scene is ensuring that it is secure. An outer perimeter is established to block public and media access, and an inner perimeter is established immediately about the scene of the rescue and the working crew. Three **control zones** are established as follows:

- Hot (coded red): This encompasses the inner perimeter and the crew as well as any area that is dangerous, such as an area contaminated by hazardous material or one in danger of a release of toxins.
- Warm (coded orange): Area for trained personnel in support of those in the hot zone. Decontamination of patients, crew, and equipment is carried out in this zone.
- Cold (coded yellow): This is the staging area and the command post (if necessary for the emergent situation). No members of the public or media should be allowed in the cold zone.

Zones are usually established by placement of police cars and fire-line tape.

The **path of least resistance** is an important concept to understand for rescues, especially if they involve fire and any products of combustion (smoke, heat, gas). Fire's path of least resistance is usually vertical and upward, although fire also spreads horizontally, especially if a vertical path is not available. It's for this reason that if there is a fire on the top floor of a building, the roof is breached to prevent horizontal spread. External factors, such as gusts of wind, can affect the path of least resistance. Water, on the other hand, also flows vertically, but downward and then

- 85 -

horizontally if the downward flow is blocked. If the EMR is rescuing patients from a building, they will often be found near the path of least resistance, such as a near a door or window. Patients should also be transported according to the path of least resistance, that is, the route that is the easiest and safest.

Multistep rescue process

The **multistep rescue process** includes the following 10 steps:

1. Preparation: Training, readying equipment, and preparing for different types of rescues.
2. Response: Using protocols for dispatch; contacting others, such as utility companies, which may have the necessary knowledge or equipment.
3. Situation size-up: 360° site survey to identify hazards and determine the need for additional personnel or equipment. Determine if the situation is rescuer/equipment intensive.
4. Stabilization: Establishing perimeters and control zones, monitoring hazardous atmosphere, carrying out lockout/tagout of industrial equipment.
5. Access: Gaining access to the patient and providing emergent care.
6. Disentanglement: Freeing the patient.
7. Removal: Continuing critical and life support while assisting the patient to move or carrying the immobilized patient. Rapid extraction if his or her condition is life threatening.
8. Transport: Transporting by various means with decontamination done as needed.
9. Scene security: Police or others providing protection of the scene, crew, and patients.
10. Postevent analysis: Reviewing the procedures performed and the problems encountered.

Occupational Safety and Health Administration (OSHA)

The **Occupational Safety and Health Administration** (OSHA) is part of the U.S. Department of Labor, and it is charged with ensuring safe, healthful working conditions and setting and enforcing workplace standards. OSHA covers most employers in the private sector, but state and federal safety regulations also generally conform to OSHA standards. Employers must provide safety training, inform workers of chemical hazards, and provide required PPE. OSHA must be notified of a workplace-related death within 8 hours and a workplace-related injury that results in hospitalization, the loss of an eye, or amputation within 24 hours. Workers may file a complaint about workplace conditions with OSHA and request an inspection. OSHA's Whistleblower Protection Program prohibits retaliation by the employer. OSHA provides Hazardous Waste Operations and Emergency Response Standard (HAZWOPER) training courses (8-hour, 24-hour, 40-hour, and refresher) for first responders. OSHA has established regulations and guidelines that are industry specific. For example, OSHA has regulations regarding EMS. OSHA requires that hazardous material be color coded, with red indicating danger; yellow, caution; orange, warning; and fluorescent orange/orange-red, biological hazard.

Hazardous materials and exposure

Hazardous materials are any that may cause harm to humans or animals by themselves or through interaction with something else. Hazardous materials may be any of the following:

- <u>Chemical:</u> Include blister agents, blood agents, choking agents, nerve agents, asphyxiants, and irritants. These can enter the body through inhalation, absorption, ingestion, and injection.
- <u>Radiological:</u> Nuclear material and radioactive substances (alpha/beta particles).
- <u>Physical/Biological:</u> Infectious wastes, blood and other body fluids, and biotoxins.

Almost any material or substance can be classified as hazardous depending on various factors such as its location, amount, and interactions. Exposure occurs when a person/animal comes in contact with the hazardous material, and contamination is the residue resulting from exposure. Absorption is the method by which hazardous material enters the bloodstream. Exposure and contamination may result in an immediate response (blistering, itching, and pain) or a delayed response (nausea, vomiting, cancer, and lung disease).

The Environmental Protection Agency (EPA) classifies **hazardous wastes** according to the following characteristics:

- Ignitable: Liquids and nonliquids that can ignite and cause fires with flash points of <60°C/140°F.
- Corrosive: Based on pH (<2 or >12.5) or its ability to corrode steel.
- Reactive: Wastes that are unstable, may react with water, or that may result in toxic gases. They may also explode.
- Toxic: Heavy metal compounds that are harmful if ingested or absorbed.

Wastes may also be classified as listed wastes. These include wastes from manufacturing and industrial processes. Hazardous wastes are often produced in manufacturing, nuclear power plants (nuclear wastes), and healthcare facilities (needles and materials contaminated with body fluids). Nuclear wastes are classified as mixed waste because they contain a radioactive component as well as a hazardous component. Hazardous wastes can result in disease (such as from needle punctures), injury (from fire and explosions), and death (from toxic exposure and disease).

The purpose of **hazardous waste site characterization** is to identify hazards and select the appropriate PPE. The team leader is responsible for the assessment, but he or she may request assistance from outside experts, such as chemists. The three steps to hazardous waste site characterization include the following:

1. Off-site characterization: Gather information/data before personnel enter the site, including the location, a description of the activities, the duration of the event, terrain information (photographs, maps), habitation/population data, accessibility, paths of least resistance, and properties of any hazardous materials/substances. Conduct the needed interviews and review of records. Perimeter reconnaissance is done with observations, air sampling, and development of a preliminary site map.
2. On-site survey: Verify the information gathered from perimeter reconnaissance, survey the area and situation, note potential exposure to hazardous materials (dust, liquid, dead animals, gas) and safety hazards (obstacles, terrain, poisonous plants), and develop a site safety plan. The entry team should have at least four members: two to enter and two for outside support who can enter the site in an emergency.
3. Ongoing monitoring: Monitoring should be continuous.

Chemical hazardous waste materials

Types of **chemical hazardous waste materials** include the following:

- Blister agents: Include sulfur mustard (mustard gas) and nitrogen mustard, which are both highly toxic. Exposure by inhalation, contact, or ingestion results in skin (erythema and blistering) and eye irritation and injury to the respiratory system as well as bone marrow suppression and gastrointestinal and neurological damage. The patient should be decontaminated within 1 to 2 minutes by flushing the eyes with water for up to 20 minutes and removing clothing and showering with soap (if available) and water for 20 minutes. Rescuers should use a self-contained breathing apparatus (SCBA), PPE (including eye protection), and chemical-protective gloves.
- Asphyxiants: Gas exposure (such as by butane, helium, and propane) lowers oxygen levels and results in suffocation. Patients require oxygen administration and may need CPR. This is especially a risk in confined spaces. Rescuers should use an SCBA.
- Blood agents: These include cyanide chloride, hydrogen cyanide, and arsine. Exposure by inhalation or ingestion. They prevent oxygen transfer from blood to cells. The patient may need oxygen and antidote. Rescuers should use an SCBA.
- Carcinogens: Agents such as asbestos, nickel compounds, and ionizing radiation that result in genetic mutation and cancer. There are various types of exposure. Patients must be removed from exposure. The rescuer must wear adequate PPE, and in some cases, he or she should use a mask or SCBA.
- Choking agents: Often, a chemical weapon is used (ammonia, chlorine) that is designed to inhibit breathing and incapacitate the person. Exposure is by inhalation, contact, or ingestion (rare). They may be corrosive to the skin and result in fluid in the lungs, leading to suffocation. Patients require supportive treatment and oxygen. Rescuers should use PPE and SCBA for most agents.
- Convulsants/Nerve agents: These include hydrazine and strychnine. Exposure may be by inhalation, contact, and ingestion. The severity of convulsions and nervous system impairment is dose related. Patients require supportive treatment. Rescuers need SCBA and protective suits (according to the exposure level of the agent).

Safety data sheets (SDSs)

Safety data sheets (SDSs), formerly known as material safety data sheets (MSDSs), explain how to handle caustic substances in the event of an accident or injury and provide pertinent information on the composition and toxic effects of chemicals in a lab. SDSs outline the proper storage of chemicals, procedures for the cleanup and dumping of caustic substances, procedures in the event of a chemical spill or injury, and the proper locations in the facility for cleanup. The SDS should also contain information indicating which substances may cause allergic effects or asthma from contact or inhalation. Emergency rescue services should obtain SDSs for common chemicals and products. Manufacturers and suppliers should have SDSs on file and can be contacted for copies. The OSHA/ Environmental Protection Agency (EPA) Occupational Chemical Database provides links for SDSs for some products. SDSs are available from various other sources, including the Toxicology Data Network (TOXNET) and poison control centers. There are also pathogen safety data sheets for biological hazards.

Multiple-casualty incidents versus mass-casualty incidents

Multiple-casualty incident	Mass-casualty incident
Involves more than one person, but different jurisdictions may quantify the total number of persons differently. Usually refers to an incident involving at least three patients. Usually involves only one jurisdiction and only one to three agencies (ambulance, fire department, and police). Requires triage, but generally only primary. Standards of care are maintained, and all patients not coded black (deceased) are transported for care.	Also involves more than one person, but may involve much larger numbers—dozens, hundreds, to thousands. Often involves multiple jurisdictions and agencies. Requires triage but may also involve separate waiting areas for color-coded individuals and secondary triage. Standards of care may be modified, and patients coded black (expectant) and not expected to live may be left in the field and/or receive delayed care if they are still living after the red- and yellow-coded individuals are transported.

Role of the transportation officer in a mass-casualty incident

During a mass-casualty event, the **transportation officer** must maintain constant communication with hospitals and trauma centers, triage officers, police, ground ambulance services, and air medical transport services. The transportation officer controls the flow of patients for treatment and must determine where to route patients in order to prevent a backlog at the receiving facility and must coordinate incoming and outgoing ambulances in the transportation staging area. The transportation officer must obtain information about each facility's surge capacity and the number and types of patients the facility is prepared to care for. The transportation officer must also coordinate air medical transport flights and determine, with the triage officer, which patients to transport by air according to their severity of injuries, availability of treatment options, and appropriate levels of care. Speed of transportation and care is often critical in a mass-casualty incident because delays often result in increased death rates.

Role of triage in a mass-casualty incident related to terrorism or a disaster

In a mass-casualty incident related to terrorism or a disaster, **rapid triage** and tagging must occur and patients must be sorted according to priority for transportation or field treatment. Because of the large numbers of casualties, triage should begin with the first patient encountered, proceeding from one to another. According to some plans, patients who are alive but expected to die are coded red, but this can result in overtriage, with too many red-coded individuals having to be transported and/or treated, resulting in patients dying during the wait. With other plans, patients expected to die are black-coded as "expectant" and left in the field or left aside until red- and yellow-coded individuals are transported and/or treated. If patients are undertriaged (such as patients who should be coded red being coded yellow instead) this can also result in increased deaths while other patients are waiting for transport and/or treatment.

Increasing survival in mass-casualty shooting and improvised explosive device incidents

Terrorist or other attacks that involve active shooters or improvised explosive devices (IEDs) often result in injuries similar to those encountered in combat situations in which the most common causes of death are extremity hemorrhage, tension pneumothorax, and airway obstruction. The **THREAT acronym** provides guidance for dealing with these situations in the following ways:

- Threat suppression: Use of police protection, ballistic vests, concealment, cover, and situational awareness. One concern is that most of the protective gear available to emergency medical personnel is for ballistics rather than explosive devices.
- Hemorrhage control: Use of tourniquets (military style) and hemostatic dressings (QuikClot) to control bleeding.
- Rapid extrication to safety: Move patients and personnel out of the danger zone to prevent further injuries.
- Assessment by medical providers: Includes provision of a nasopharyngeal airway or upright seating and leaning forward for airway compromise and spinal precautions.
- Transport to definitive care: Medical treatment should continue during transport.

Safety issues associated with active shooters and terrorist bomb attacks

With **active shooters,** standard protocol has been for emergency response services to wait until the police have removed the threat and secured the area before moving in to care for victims; however, this delay in treatment may result in death, so some authorities are now recommending that emergency response personnel enter the scene with police while wearing appropriate protective equipment, although this does pose some risk, especially with additional shooters or a secondary attack. With a **terrorist bombing** and improvised explosive devices (IEDs), situational awareness is critical because multiple explosive devices (some undetonated) may be at the scene. IEDs may be inside backpacks, suitcases, and packages left unattended, but in emergency situations, innocent people often drop backpacks and packages and run away. Additionally, attackers wearing suicide vests or belts may mix in with other victims or people escaping the blast area.

Bomb threat standoff recommendations

Threat	Explosive capacity (lb)	Mandatory evacuation distance (ft)	Preferred evacuation distance (ft)	Shelter-in-place zone (ft)
Pipe bomb	5	70	1200+	71–1199
Suicide bomber	20	110	1700+	111–1699
Suitcase /Briefcase	50	150	1850+	151–1849
Automobile	500	320	1900+	321–1899
SUV/Van	1000	400	2400+	401–2399
Small truck	4000	640	3800+	641–3799
Container truck	10,000	860	5100+	861–5099
Semitrailer	60,000	1570	9300+	1571–9299

Source: U.S. Department of Homeland Security.

B-NICE hazardous material (hazmat) incidents associated with terrorist attacks

Category	Response
B—Biological (bacteria, viruses, fungi, toxins)	Inhalation type—evacuate for 80 feet, shut down air-handling systems, wear appropriate PPE and SCBA, and avoid contamination. Visible agent—decontaminate with soap and water. Symptoms may vary but are usually delayed.
N—Nuclear/ Radiological	Inhalation type (most common)—Isolate/Secure the area, avoid smoke/fumes, stay upwind, and use PPE and SCBA. Isolate victims and decontaminate as appropriate. Symptoms are usually delayed.
I—Incendiary	Be on alert for multiple devices and sabotaged fire suppression equipment. Symptoms include burns, pain, and trauma.
C—Chemical	Isolate/Secure the area, decontaminate victims with soap and water, and be on alert for chemical dispersal devices. Approach toward uphill and upwind. Isolate symptomatic patients from others. Symptoms vary but may include burns, blistering, vomiting, breathing difficulty, and neurological damage.
E—Explosives	Be alert for secondary devices, undetonated devices, and secondary hazards (unstable buildings and debris). Remove victims from the area, secure the perimeter, and stage away from the incident area. Decontaminate as necessary. Symptoms include burns, amputations, cuts, and penetrating and blunt trauma.

"All-hazards" safety approach to mass-casualty incidents

The **"all-hazards" safety approach** to mass-casualty incidents aims to provide plans that can be used to deal with all types of hazards (natural disasters, terrorist attacks, and mass-casualty incidents) as well as encompassing the four components of emergency management: mitigation, preparedness, response, and recovery. Organizations in an area coordinate to develop joint action plans that can be activated in response to incidents, with the chain of command clearly outlined. This approach lowers costs to individual organizations and provides for faster and more effective response. However, although the basic structure may be the same for responding to all hazards, there are inevitable differences between (for example) a terrorist attack with active shooters and a natural disaster, such as a hurricane, which can be anticipated and mitigated to some degree. For this reason, modifying existing incident action plans to meet the needs of a situation is essential.

Treating terrorists and criminals

In mass-casualty incidents, **terrorists and criminals** involved in the incident may be injured and require treatment, and EMS personnel may feel conflicted about providing treatment when others have been injured or killed, but it's important to provide treatment to terrorists and criminals the same as any other individuals because (1) they are in need of help and (2) their survival may be critical to identifying coconspirators and to providing reasons for the attack. However, these individuals may pose risks to emergency medical personnel, so they should be examined while under police guard. The individual's hands should be examined first to check for weapons and detonators and secured (with handcuffs, if possible). Clothes should be examined and removed very carefully in case the person is wearing a suicide device of some type. Emergency medical personnel should also be aware that the individual may be feigning injury or unconsciousness.

EMR Practice Test

1. The best strategy for assessing a 2-year-old child is to:

   a. touch the head first.
   b. remove the child's clothing.
   c. have the parent hold the child.
   d. have the child examined by an EMR of the same gender.

2. Which of the following statements regarding the fontanelles in infants is false?

   a. The fontanelles may bulge when the infant is crying.
   b. The fontanelles may pulsate with each heartbeat.
   c. The fontanelles at the top of the head does not close until 18 months of age.
   d. The fontanelles at the top of the head closes at 10 months of age.

3. Compared with adults, infants:

   a. primarily breathe through the mouth.
   b. primarily breathe through the nose.
   c. breathe through the mouth when the nasal airway is obstructed.
   d. have more respiratory movement in the chest.

4. Blood pressure is higher in:

   a. females.
   b. males.
   c. shorter children.
   d. inactive children.

5. In the case of an infant with SIDS, the EMR should do all of the following except:

   a. attempt to diagnose SIDS.
   b. provide resuscitation to the infant.
   c. comfort the parents.
   d. arrange for transport of the infant to a hospital.

6. Treatment of a child with a fever should include:

   a. application of rubbing alcohol.
   b. undressing the child.
   c. bundling up the child.
   d. bathing the child in cold water.

7. In an MCI, the EMR is expected to:

   a. triage as many patients as possible.
   b. provide care to as many patients as possible.
   c. provide care to the walking wounded.
   d. take copious notes on each patient.

8. According to the START triage system, patients are classified as delayed if:

   a. he/she is able to walk away.
   b. he/she is unable to follow commands.
   c. their radial pulse is absent.
   d. capillary refill is <2 seconds.

9. In triage, a red tag indicates:

    a. nonsalvageable status.
    b. immediate status.
    c. delayed status.
    d. deteriorated status.

10. Which of the following statements regarding assessment of the circulatory system in children during triage is false?

    a. A nonbreathing child may still have a pulse.
    b. In children, respiratory failure is followed by circulatory failure.
    c. Small children have a respiratory rate >30 breaths per minute.
    d. A respiratory rate of 8 breaths per minute in a child is normal.

11. According to the JumpSTART triage system,:

    a. a nonbreathing child is classified as deceased.
    b. a nonbreathing child should be assessed for a pulse.
    c. a child who responds appropriately to pain is classified as immediate.
    d. a child who breathes spontaneously after ventilation is classified as delayed.

12. All of the following statements regarding the palpation method of obtaining blood pressure are false except:

    a. palpation measures only diastolic blood pressure.
    b. A stethoscope is used for palpation.
    c. palpation measures only systolic blood pressure.
    d. Palpation is more accurate than auscultation.

13. The systolic blood pressure of an adult male is measured by:

    a. adding the age to 90.
    b. adding the age to 100.
    c. dividing the diastolic measurement by two thirds.
    d. multiplying the age in years by 2 and adding 80.

14. In measuring blood pressure using the auscultation method,:

    a. readings should be rounded off to the next highest number.
    b. the last fade of sound should be used as the systolic pressure.
    c. the systolic pressure is indicated when the sound becomes dull or soft.
    d. the first significant sound heard is the diastolic pressure.

15. The blow-by oxygenation method is used in:

    a. patients with chronic obstructive pulmonary disease (COPD).
    b. premature infants.
    c. elderly patients.
    d. asthma patients.

16. High-flow oxygen can cause respiratory arrest in:

    a. preterm infants.
    b. COPD patients.
    c. elderly patients.
    d. pediatric patients.

17. All of the following are types of COPD except:

   a. emphysema.
   b. bronchitis.
   c. asthma.
   d. black lung disease.

18. Which of the following statements regarding hyperventilation is false?

   a. Hyperventilation may result in cyanosis.
   b. Hyperventilation may be a sign of a heart attack.
   c. Hyperventilation may be resolved by reassuring the patient.
   d. Hyperventilation may be treated by having the patient blow into a paper bag.

19. Low blood sugar may be associated with:

   a. stroke.
   b. COPD.
   c. altered mental status.
   d. cerebrovascular accident.

20. Ketone breath is a sign of:

   a. hypoglycemia.
   b. hyperglycemia.
   c. cyanosis.
   d. COPD.

21. Which of the following statements regarding hypoglycemia is false?

   a. Hypoglycemia may resemble alcohol intoxication.
   b. Hypoglycemic patients may be given honey, candy, or a soft drink.
   c. Hypoglycemia may result from a diabetic not taking insulin.
   d. Hypoglycemia may result in ketone breath.

22. The first step in treating a victim of ingested poisoning should be to:

   a. dilute the poison.
   b. administer activated charcoal.
   c. give the patient a glass of water.
   d. contact a poison control center.

23. A pocket face mask with a HEPA filter may be required to treat ingestion of:

   a. ammonia.
   b. arsenic.
   c. kerosene.
   d. gasoline.

24. Treatment of a bee sting should include all of the following, except:

   a. the administration of oxygen.
   b. taking body substance isolation (BSI) precautions.
   c. scraping away the stinger.
   d. pulling out the stinger.

25. Which of the following statements regarding heat stroke is false?

    a. Heat stroke may be life-threatening.
    b. Heat stroke patients usually present with altered mental status.
    c. Heat stroke patients perspire heavily.
    d. The skin of a heat stroke patient is hot to the touch.

26. All of the following are accepted practices in the treatment of heat exhaustion, except:

    a. the application of ice bags to the neck, armpits, and groin.
    b. giving the patient a glass of water.
    c. loosening or removing the patient's clothing.
    d. providing oxygen.

27. Which of the following statements regarding generalized cold emergencies is true?

    a. Hypothermia only occurs when the outside temperature is below freezing.
    b. Cold emergency victims may show no vital signs but may still be revived.
    c. Cold emergency patients should be given hot tea or coffee to warm up.
    d. Cold emergency patients should be encouraged to walk to warm up.

28. Emergency care of a late-localized cold injury includes:

    a. massage of the injured area.
    b. the application of heat to the injured area.
    c. walking to stimulate circulation.
    d. covering the injured area.

29. Emergency care of a patient with a behavioral emergency includes:

    a. the placement of the patient on the cot and the application of restraints.
    b. playing along with hallucinations.
    c. asking the patient what is troubling him or her.
    d. obtaining the patient's consent to provide care.

30. Emergency care of drug abuse or overdose patients involves:

    a. asking the patient if he or she is using drugs.
    b. performing a physical examination.
    c. memorizing drug names and reactions.
    d. reassuring the patient.

31. Which of the following statements regarding cardiac compromise is false?

    a. Damage over an electrical pathway may cause cardiac arrest.
    b. Most cardiac arrests result from myocardial infarction (MI).
    c. Most MIs result in cardiac arrest.
    d. A heart attack is not the same thing as a cardiac arrest.

32. Angina pectoris is:
    a. damaging to the heart muscles.
    b. the same thing as a heart attack.
    c. treated the same as a heart attack.
    d. a backup of fluid within the circulatory system.

33. All of the following are signs and symptoms of congestive heart failure (CHF), except:

    a. fatigue.

→ b. slowed pulse rate.

    c. edema.

    d. jugular venous distention (JVD).

34. Sacral edema is a symptom of:

    a. angina.

    b. MI.

→ c. CHF.

    d. COPD.

35. All of the following may be used to treat an acute angina attack, except:

→ a. nitroglycerin patches.

    b. aspirin.

    c. nitroglycerin spray.

    d. nitroglycerin tablets.

36. The OPQRST mnemonic may also be used to assess:

    a. altered mental status.

→ b. shortness of breath.

    c. stroke.

    d. hyperglycemia.

37. Moving a patient is necessary in all of the following situations, except:

    a. to assess ABCs.

    b. to assess bleeding.

    c. to gain access to other patients.

→ d. to treat neck pain.

38. Which of the following emergency moves requires more than one rescuer?

    a. Piggyback carry

→ b. Extremity lift

    c. Pack-strap carry

    d. Firefighter's carry

39. The direct ground lift is typically performed by ___ rescuer(s).

    a. two

→ b. three

    c. one

    d. four

40. Which of the following is NOT recommended as a primary spinal immobilization device?

→ a. Scoop stretcher

    b. Vest-type extrication device

    c. Pedi-board

    d. Backboard

41. The drag method may be used to move patients in all of the following cases, except:

    a. when the patient is unresponsive.
    b. when the patient has a suspected spinal injury.
→ c. when the situation is not urgent.
    d. when the scene is hazardous.

42. Which of the following is an example of an emergency move?

    a. Extremity lift
→ b. Drag method
    c. Direct ground lift
    d. Draw sheet method

43. The thorax encompasses the:

    a. abdomen.
    b. pelvic cavity.
→ c. chest.
    d. mandible.

44. A patient in the lateral recumbent position is resting on his or her:

    a. back.
→ b. side.
    c. stomach.
    d. elbow.

45. The first priority of an EMR in a violent or dangerous situation is to:

→ a. ensure personal safety.
    b. ensure patient safety.
    c. disburse onlookers.
    d. assess the patient's ABCs.

46. Which of the following statements regarding patient consent is false?

    a. Children cannot give consent.
→ b. Consent must always be verbal.
    c. A mentally ill patient is subject to implied consent.
    d. A DNR order may be in the form of a bracelet.

47. All of the following statements regarding legal issues of patient care are false, except:

    a. the scope of practice defines the type of care a patient should receive.
    b. the standard of care remains the same regardless of local law.
    c. suicidal patients who respond to questions are competent to give consent.
→ d. a patient does not have to speak to refuse care.

48. Which of the following may protect an EMR from civil liability?

    a. DNR order
    b. Scope of practice
→ c. Good Samaritan law
    d. Duty to act

49. Patient confidentiality does NOT apply in all of the following cases, except:

    a. elder abuse.

→ b. other EMR personnel .

    c. healthcare providers involved in the patient's care.

    d. rape.

50. Airway obstruction may be caused by all of the following, except:

→ a. asthma.

    b. burns.

    c. bee sting.

✗ d. infection.

51. Which of the following statements regarding breathing is false?

    a. Clinical death can be reversed.

→ b. Biological death can be reversed.

    c. A pH imbalance may cause respiratory failure.

    d. Biological death results when too many brain cells die.

52. Which of the following is used to open the airway of a patient with a spinal injury?

    a. Head-tilt, chin-lift maneuver

    b. Mouth-to-mouth procedure

→ c. Jaw-thrust maneuver

    d. Mouth-to-nose procedure

53. Abdominal thrusts to clear the airway of a choking individual may be:

    a. used on children under 1 year of age.

→ b. given by straddling the legs of the patient.

    c. used on pregnant women.

    d. used on obese patients.

54. Which of the following statements regarding airway adjuncts is false?

    a. The oropharyngeal airway (OPA), nasopharyngeal airway (NPA), and bag-valve-mask (BVM) may be used together.

    b. OPAs may only be used on patients without a gag reflex.

    c. NPAs are preferred for patients with a gag reflex.

→ d. It is not necessary to maintain an open airway when using an OPA.

55. The NPA should NOT be used in:

    a. responsive patients

    b. infants.

→ c. patients with facial fractures.

    d. patients with a gag reflex.

56. The ___may be used to gauge the size of a patient's nostril opening.

→ a. little finger

    b. index finger

    c. earlobe

    d. thumb

57. If the NPA will not advance into the nostril, the EMR should do all of the following, except:

a. insert the NPA into the opposite nostril.

b. use an airway that is smaller in diameter.

c. use petroleum jelly to lubricate the outside of the tube.

d. use scissors to change the bevel.

58. Which of the following statements regarding the insertion of an airway is false?

a. Elderly patients are prone to nosebleeds while placing an NPA.

b. The BVM should be placed before inserting an NPA.

c. The BVM is an effective infection-control barrier.

d. The BVM may be used for drug overdose patients.

59. All of the following statements regarding suctioning are true, except:

a. suctioning also removes oxygen from the airway.

b. finger sweeps may be used to remove fluid and other matter from the oral cavity.

c. suctioning should be performed for no more than 15 seconds.

d. the tip of the catheter should be placed directly over the back of the tongue.

60. The mechanism of injury (MOI) should be assessed in:

a. responsive medical patients.

b. unresponsive medical patients.

c. trauma patients.

d. elderly patients.

61. In the scene size-up of a medical patient, the EMR should do all of the following, except:

a. evaluate the nature of illness (NOI).

b. take BSI precautions.

c. evaluate scene safety.

d. evaluate the need for spinal immobilization.

62. The ABCs of emergency care are used to assess:

a. mental status.

b. pediatric patients.

c. immediate threats to life.

d. MOI.

63. The verbal component of the AVPU scale means that:

a. the patient initiated a conversation.

b. the patient answered questions.

c. the patient responded to a loud verbal stimulus.

d. the patient was unresponsive.

64. In a small child, the pulse is typically taken at the:

a. wrist.

b. neck.

c. finger.

d. arm.

65. In assessing an infant, the EMR should:

   a. tilt the head back to open the airway.

→ b. flick the bottom of the infant's feet.

   c. grasp the wrist to take a pulse.

   d. take the blood pressure.

66. Priority dispatching of EMS involves all of the following, except:

   a. determining the need for advanced life support (ALS).

   b. determining the need for basic life support (BLS).

   c. determining response mode.

→ d. determining a focused history.

67. In patient assessment, subjective findings refer to:

   a. signs.

→ b. symptoms.

   c. vital signs.

   d. ABCs.

68. Which of the following statements regarding obtaining a patient history is false?

   a. The patient history and physical examination can be performed together.

   b. The patient history can be obtained while treating a bleeding wound.

→ c. Vital signs should not be taken until after the history is obtained.

   d. When obtaining a patient history, the term "drugs" should not be used.

69. All of the following questions may be asked as part of the SAMPLE history, except:

→ a. how old are you?

   b. are you taking any medication(s)?

   c. when did you last eat?

   d. what happened?

70. A rapid, weak pulse may indicate:

   a. stroke.

   b. cardiac arrest.

→ c. shock.

   d. high blood pressure.

71. Both a rapid, strong pulse and a rapid, weak pulse can be associated with:

   a. stroke.

→ b. heat emergency.

   c. high blood pressure.

   d. low blood pressure.

72. Which of the following statements regarding the radial pulse isfalse?

   a. A radial pulse may be undetectable if the patient has low blood pressure.

   b. A radial pulse may be undetectable if the patient has an injury to an extremity.

→ c. CPR should be started if the radial pulse is absent.

   d. The thumb should not be used to take a radial pulse.

73. Snoring is most often associated with:

    a. stroke.
    b. asthma. - wheezing
    c. fractured rib. blood
    d. pneumonia. Shallow
                    breathing

74. Skin color, temperature, and moisture may be assessed at all of the following sites, except the:

    a. abdomen.
    b. cheek.
    c. forehead.
    d. extremities.

75. A cyanotic skin color may indicate:

    a. decreased blood pressure.
    b. inadequate heart function.
    c. shock.
    d. emotional distress.

76. Jaundiced skin is a sign of:

    a. shock.
    b. carbon monoxide poisoning.
    c. liver abnormalities.
    d. vitamin deficiency.

77. Anxiety may be indicated by:

    a. hot, moist skin.
    b. goose bumps.
    c. cold, dry skin.
    d. cool, clammy skin.

78. Unequal pupils may indicate:

    a. reaction to medication.
    b. head injury.
    c. shock.
    d. damage to the central nervous system.

79. In the acronym BP-DOC, "C" stands for:

    a. contusions.
    b. confusion.
    c. crepitus.
    d. convulsions.

80. In the acronym DCAP-BTLS, "B" stands for:

    a. bruising.
    b. bleeding.
    c. brain injury.
    d. burns.

81. The dorsalis pedis pulse is located lateral to the:
    a. ankle.
    b. big toe.
    c. thumb.
    d. wrist.

82. The posterior tibial pulse may be taken:
    a. behind the ankle.
    b. lateral to the big toe.
    c. at the wrist.
    d. at the top of the foot.

83. The memory aid OPQRST may be used to assess the:
    a. trauma patient with no significant MOI.
    b. unresponsive medical patient.
    c. responsive medical patient.
    d. trauma patient with significant MOI.

84. In the acronym OPQRST, "R" stands for:
    a. respirations.
    b. region and radiate.
    c. râles.
    d. rate.

85. Which of the following statements regarding CPR technique in a child is false?
    a. The rate of compressions is the same as in adults.
    b. For one-rescuer CPR, the rate of compressions to breaths is the same as in adults.
    c. The depth of compressions is the same as in adults.
    d. The mouth-to-barrier device may be used in both adults and children.

86. CPR may be stopped under all of the following circumstances, except:
    a. when the patient regains a pulse.
    b. when the patient regains breathing.
    c. when you are too tired to continue.
    d. when the patient has no pulse.

87. Which of the following statements regarding one-rescuer CPR is false?
    a. An adult patient may be left alone while calling for help.
    b. CPR should be performed on a child for 2 minutes before calling for help.
    c. A bystander should not be allowed to perform CPR.
    d. A bystander may be allowed to perform chest compressions.

88. Which of the following statements regarding two-rescuer CPR is false?
    a. Either rescuer may request a change of positions if he or she is tired.
    b. The ventilator should decide when to change positions.
    c. The compressor should decide when to change positions.
    d. The compressor should complete 30 compressions before changing positions.

- 102 -

89. A cracking sound heard during chest compression indicates:
    a. proper chest compression.
    b. fractured ribs.
    c. excess air in the lungs.
    d. excess air in the stomach.

90. CPR may be stopped when:
    a. the physician at the scene orders you to stop.
    b. the patient's family has requested that you discontinue.
    c. the patient is in cardiac arrest.
    d. the patient has a terminal illness.

91. An automated external defibrillator (AED) is NOT effective in the case of:
    a. ventricular tachycardia.
    b. shock.
    c. asystole.
    d. ventricular fibrillation.

92. An AED should NOT be placed on a patient who is:
    a. unresponsive.
    b. younger than 1 year.
    c. without a pulse.
    d. not breathing.

93. Which of the following statements regarding proper placement of an AED is false?
    a. An AED may be placed on a patient lying on a wet surface.
    b. An AED should not be placed in a moving ambulance.
    c. An AED may be placed on a patient lying in a puddle of water.
    d. An AED should not be placed on a patient with an obstructed airway.

94. When operating a fully automated defibrillator, the EMR should do all of the following, except:
    a. begin CPR before setting up the defibrillator.
    b. begin CPR following the shock.
    c. begin CPR if the patient goes into a rhythm that is not shockable.
    d. continue CPR with the defibrillator attached if the patient does not have a pulse.

95. In an adult male patient, a blood loss of ___would be considered lethal.
    a. 6.6 liters
    b. 2.2 liters
    c. 1.5 liters
    d. 30 milliliters

96. The flow of blood is slow in the case of:
    a. venous bleeding.
    b. arterial bleeding.
    c. capillary bleeding.
    d. external bleeding.

97. In the case of ___ bleeding, the color of the blood may appear dark maroon.

    a. capillary
    • b. venous
    c. arterial
    d. abdominal

98. The first step in controlling external bleeding is:

    a. elevation.
    b. pressure points.
    •c. applying direct pressure.
    d. applying a tourniquet.

99. Elevation with direct pressure should be used to control bleeding in the case of:

    a. fractures.
    b. impaled objects.
    c. spinal injury.
    → d. leg injury.

100. In an elderly patient, the most reliable sign of shock from internal bleeding is:

    a. rapid breathing.
    b. weak pulse.
    • c. level of consciousness.
    d. dilated pupils.

Answer Key and Explanations

1. C: Toddlers, or children one to three years of age, should be examined in a head-to-toe manner, as touching the head first may frighten the child. Toddlers do not wish to be separated from their parents; thus, the child should be held by a parent during the examination. Because toddlers dislike having clothing removed, only one article of clothing should be removed at a time and replaced immediately after examination. It is not necessary for the EMR to be the same gender as the child; however, in the case of an adolescent, the physical examination should be conducted by an EMR of the same gender.

2. D: The fontanelles, or soft spots on the head of an infant, may bulge when the infant is crying or agitated and may pulsate with each heartbeat; thus, they should only be assessed when the infant is quiet. The largest soft spot, located on the top of the infant's head, does not close completely until the infant is approximately 18 months of age.

3. B: Compared with adults, infants primarily breathe through the nose; thus, unlike adults, when the nasal airway is obstructed, infants do not automatically breathe through the mouth. Because the diaphragm is the major breathing muscle in the infant, more respiratory movement is seen in the abdomen than in the chest.

4. B: In children, blood pressure is dependent upon gender, age, and height. Blood pressure is higher in males than in females, as well as in taller children vs shorter children. Blood pressure is higher in children engaged in exercise or activity than in inactive children.

5. A: Because the EMR cannot diagnose sudden infant death syndrome (SIDS), he or she should provide the infant with the same emergency care as a patient in cardiac arrest. The EMR should provide resuscitation and arrange transport of the infant to the hospital; however, resuscitation should not be attempted if rigor mortis has developed or the infant's blood has pooled: Emotional support should be given to the parents.

6. B: Bundling up a child with a fever simply retains the heat of the fever and is therefore ineffective; instead, the child should be undressed to his or her underwear or diaper. If the child becomes chilled, he or she should be covered with a light blanket. Applying rubbing alcohol may allow toxic amounts to be absorbed through the skin. Children with fever should never be submerged in cold water.

7. A: In the case of a multiple-casualty incident (MCI), EMR personnel are the first on the scene and are responsible for triaging as many patients as possible; triage should only be stopped when a patient requires life-saving care. Patients with minor injuries, or the walking wounded, should be directed to a location away from the scene of the emergency. Brief notes should be taken on each patient; however, taking copious notes may delay the triage process.

8. D: According to the START triage system, a patient is classified as delayed if respirations are <30 per minute, capillary refill is <2 seconds or radial pulse is present, and the patient is able to follow commands. Patients who are the least injured and are able to walk away from the scene are classified as minor.

9. B: In triage, a red tag indicates immediate status; such patients are unresponsive but able to breathe. Non-salvageable or deceased status is indicated by a black or gray tag and delayed status by a yellow tag.

10. D: In children, circulatory failure follows respiratory failure; thus, a nonbreathing child may still have a pulse. Small children, particularly infants, have a respiratory rate >30 breaths per minute. According to the START triage system, a respiratory rate of <30 breaths per minute in an adult is a positive sign; thus, a child with a respiratory rate <8 breaths per minute would be classified as delayed when he or she is actually in respiratory failure.

11. B: According to the JumpSTART triage system, a nonbreathing child should be assessed for a pulse; if the child does not begin to breathe spontaneously after the airway is opened, he or she should be ventilated five times. If the child begins to breathe spontaneously after ventilation, he or she should be classified as immediate. A child who is alert and responds appropriately to pain should be classified as delayeD.

12. C: The palpation method of obtaining blood pressure involves using a blood pressure cuff and feeling the patient's radial or brachial pulse. Palpation only reveals systolic blood pressure and is not as accurate as the auscultation method, which uses both a blood pressure cuff and a stethoscope and measures both diastolic and systolic blood pressure.

13. B: The systolic blood pressure in adult males is measured by adding the age to 100; in women, systolic blood pressure is measured by adding the age to 90. In children, the systolic blood pressure is measured by multiplying the age by 2 and adding 80. Diastolic blood pressure is two thirds that of the systolic measurement.

14. A: In measuring blood pressure using the auscultation method, readings should be rounded off to the next highest number. The first significant sound heard is the systolic blood pressure; as the cuff deflates, dulling or softening of the sound indicates diastolic pressure. The last fade of sound indicates the diastolic pressure.

15. B: Oxygen should only be administered directly to a newborn infant under certain circumstances, such as premature or difficult delivery or respiratory distress. The blow-by method in which the mask is placed near the side of the nose and mouth may be useful in infants.

16. B: Because patients with COPD have a hypoxic drive, or are accustomed to having lower levels of oxygen in the lungs and blood, prolonged use of high-flow oxygen may lower the drive to breathe, resulting in respiratory arrest. High-flow oxygen may cause eye damage in premature infants.

17. C: Emphysema, chronic bronchitis, and black lung disease are all types of COPD.

18. D: Hyperventilation is uncontrolled, rapid, deep breathing that may occur in association with anxiety, fear, or stress. Although most cases are self-correcting, hyperventilation may be a sign of a more serious medical condition such as respiratory distress or impending heart attack; patients may experience cyanosis, or bluish discoloration of the skin, lips, and nail beds. Hyperventilation may be treated by simply reassuring the patient and having him or her take slow, deep breaths. Contrary to popular belief, hyperventilation should not be treated by having the patient blow into a paper bag.

19. C: Low blood sugar or diabetes is associated with altered mental status; altered mental status may result from seizures, cardiac events, and stroke, or cerebrovascular accident.

20. B: Ketones have an odor resembling acetone, or nail polish remover. Ketone breath, or breath with a sweet or fruity odor, is a sign of hyperglycemia.

21. C: Hypoglycemia, or insulin shock, may result from a diabetic taking too much insulin; hyperglycemia, or diabetic coma, results when a diabetic does not take his or her insulin. Hypoglycemia may produce abnormal, hostile, or aggressive behavior resembling that associated with alcohol intoxication; patients may be given oral glucose or a sugar substitute such as honey, candy, or a soft drink. Ketone breath is a sign of hyperglycemia.

22. D: In the case of ingested poisoning, the EMR should first call the poison control center; no care should be provided other than the ABCs to control life-threatening situations. Providing liquids to a patient who has ingested poison may be dangerous.

23. B: In the case of a patient who has ingested a highly concentrated dose of arsenic, cyanide, or another poison that may leave a deposit on the patient's lips, use of a pocket face mask with a HEPA filter, a bag-valve mask, or other protective barrier device may be required to protect the EMR from exposure.

24. D: In treating a patient who has been stung by a bee or wasp, the EMR should first perform scene size-up, including taking BSI precautions. Oxygen should be administered and the stinger should be scraped away from, not pulled out of, the patient's skin.

25. C: Heat stroke is a life-threatening condition; signs and symptoms include altered mental status, skin that is hot to the touch, and convulsions. Heavy perspiration is a sign of heat exhaustion.

26. A: In treating a patient with heat exhaustion, he or she should first be moved to a cool place; the patient's clothing should be loosened or removed and oxygen provided as per local protocol. If the patient is responsive, he or she may be given a glass of water; however, the patient should not be chilled. In treating heat stroke, which is considered a life-threatening condition, the patient should be cooled as rapidly as possible; applying cold packs or ice bags to the neck, armpits, and groin is effective in rapidly cooling a patient with heat stroke.

27. B: Hypothermia can still occur if the outside temperature is above freezing. Although a generalized cold emergency victim may be unresponsive and show no vital signs, it should not be assumed that he or she is dead; the pulse should be assessed for 30 to 45 seconds, and CPR begun if there is still no pulse. Giving the patient hot coffee or tea or alcoholic beverages may affect the blood vessels and worsen his or her condition. Patients should be removed from the cold environment, but should not be allowed to walk or exert themselves.

28. D: In the case of a late-localized cold injury, the injured area should be covered and should not be re-exposed to cold. The EMR should not attempt to rub or massage or apply heat to the injured area; patients should not be allowed to walk on affected legs.

29. C: In the case of a behavioral emergency, the EMR should perform a scene size-up and consider the need for law enforcement. Behavioral emergency patients often refuse to consent to care; thus, medical direction should always be consulted before attempting to provide emergency care. Potentially violent patients should not be restrained unless directed by medical direction and/or law enforcement. Playing along with the patient's visual or auditory hallucinations or arguing or challenging the patient is not acceptable. Instead, acknowledge that the patient is upset and ask what is troubling him or her in a calm, reassuring voice.

30. D: Emergency care of a drug abuse or overdose patient is basically the same regardless of the drug used and should not change unless ordered by medical direction or the poison control center. Memorizing specific drug names and reactions is unnecessary. Because many drug abusers use more than one drug, performing a physical examination is not helpful in detecting which drugs have

caused the problem. Instead, life support should be provided and vital signs should be monitored; oxygen should be administered according to local protocols. Most drug abuse patients will not provide information about their drug use; asking the patient if he or she is taking medications rather than drugs may elicit a better response. Talk to the patient and reassure him or her throughout all phases of care.

31. C: A heart attack, or MI, is not the same thing as a cardiac arrest. Most cardiac arrests result from MIs; however, most MIs do not result in cardiac arrest. Damage over an important electrical pathway or damage to the left ventricle may result in cardiac arrest.

32. C: Angina pectoris is chest pain caused by an insufficient supply of blood to the heart muscle; however, it does do cause any damage to the heart muscle. Although it is not the same thing as a heart attack, the signs and symptoms of angina are identical to those of a heart attack; thus, patients with cardiac-related pain should be treated in the same manner as a heart attack victim. CHF is a condition in which the heart cannot adequately circulate blood, resulting in a backup of fluid in the lungs and other organs.

33. B: The signs and symptoms of CHF include shortness of breath, chest discomfort, rapid pulse rate, pedal or sacral edema, and JVD; elderly patients may also complain of fatigue.

34. C: Sacral edema, or swelling of the sacral areas of the body, is a symptom of CHF; it is often seen in patients confined to bed and results when gravity pulls excess fluid in the lungs and other areas downward.

35. A: Angina patients typically have prescriptions for nitroglycerin tablets or spray; placing a tablet or spraying one dose under the patient's tongue allows the drug to rapidly enter the bloodstream; however, transdermal nitroglycerin patches are prescribed to prevent and not treat angina and are too slow to be of use in treating an acute angina attack. Aspirin is commonly used to treat suspected heart attack.

36. B: The mnemonic OPQRST stands for Onset, Provocation, Quality, Region and Radiate, Severity, and Time; it is often used to assess chest pain and may also be used to assess shortness of breath. The AVPU scale is used to assess altered mental status.

37. D: Moving a patient should be avoided unless it is absolutely necessary; patients should be moved only when ABCs or bleeding cannot be assessed adequately, when the patient is in a dangerous environment or at risk for further injury, or when access to other patients needing life-saving care cannot be obtained. Avoid moving patients with neck pain, weakness, or numbness to prevent the risk of spinal injury.

38. B: The piggyback carry, firefighter's carry, and pack-strap carry may all be performed by one rescuer; the extremity lift involves moving a patient from the ground or chair to a chair or stretcher, and requires two rescuers.

39. B: The direct ground lift involves moving a patient from the ground or floor to a bed or stretcher; although two rescuers can perform this move, three are recommended.

40. A: The long spine board or backboard is used for patients with a suspected spinal injury who are found lying down or standing; the vest-type extrication device is used to extricate a seated patient while stabilizing the head, neck, and spine. The Pedi-board is a special spinal immobilization board used for infants and children. The scoop stretcher is typically used for patients with hip or multiple injuries and is not recommended for patients with spinal injuries.

41. C: The drag method is an emergency move that may be performed when the scene is hazardous, when the patient needs immediate repositioning, or when you must reach another patient requiring life-saving care; it is recommended for heavy or unresponsive patients or those who are unable to move or with suspected spinal injuries.

42. B: The extremity lift, direct ground lift, and draw sheet method are all useful in moving patients in a nonemergency situation; the drag method is used when the scene is hazardous, when the patient requires immediate repositioning, or in order to reach another patient who requires life-saving care.

43. C: The torso encompasses the abdomen, chest, or thorax, and the pelvic cavity; the mandible is otherwise known as the lower jaw.

44. B: A patient lying on his or her side is in the lateral recumbent position; a supine patient is lying face up and a prone patient face down.

45. A: The first priority for an EMR in a violent or dangerous situation, even before patient care, is to ensure his or her own safety; the EMR should not enter a scene until he or she is certain it is safe.

46. B: Patient consent may be nonverbal; by not pulling away or stopping the EMR from providing care, the patient is giving consent. Mentally ill or developmentally challenged patients or patients experiencing a behavioral emergency may receive care under implied consent, which assumes that the patient's caregiver would give consent for treatment. Legally, children cannot refuse care or give consent; only a parent or guardian can give consent. A DNR, or Do Not Resuscitate order, is not just the expressed consent of the patient or family but is an actual legal document; some patients may wear a DNR bracelet.

47. D: The scope of practice refers to what is legally permitted to be done by an EMR; however, it does not define what type of care a particular patient should receive in specific situations. The standard of care is the type of care that should be provided based on local law, administrative orders, and local guidelines and protocols. Asking questions such as where the patient is, the of day or month, or what has happened to the patient are useful in determining a patient's competency; however, in the case of a suicidal patient, answering questions correctly does not necessarily mean he or she is competent to consent to or refuse care. Refusal of care may be nonverbal; shaking the head to indicate "no" or holding up a hand to indicate "stop" are also regarded as refusal of care.

48. C: A DNR order is a legal document stating that the patient has a terminal illness and does not want to be resuscitated. The scope of practice refers to what is legally permitted for an EMR to do; the duty to act is the legal requirement that an EMR must provide care according to standard operating procedures. All EMR personnel are trained to deliver the standard of care specific to their locality; in some states, Good Samaritan laws protect EMR personnel from civil liability if they have delivered care in good faith and to the level of their training and ability.

49. B: Patient confidentiality refers to the treatment of information disclosed by a patient; information such as the name of the patient, statements the patient might have made, or descriptions of the patient's behavior or personal appearance should not be shared with anyone except other healthcare providers involved in the continued care of the patient. Patient confidentiality does not apply in cases of rape, elder or child abuse, or if the EMR receives a subpoena to testify in court.

50. A: Airway obstruction may be caused by tissue damage, such as upper airway burns resulting from breathing hot air in a fire, allergic reactions, such as a bee sting, and epiglottic or pharyngeal

infections. A common symptom of asthma is wheezing, resulting from swelling or spasm along the lower airway; however, wheezing is not usually associated with airway obstruction.

51. B: Clinical death, or the moment when both breathing and heartbeat stop, may be reversed if CPR is given within 10 minutes; biological death occurs when too many brain cells die and cannot be reversed. If blood pH is either too high or low, brain functions, including those that affect breathing, may cease.

52. C: The jaw-thrust procedure is used to open the airway of a patient with a suspected spinal injury; the head-tilt, chin-lift maneuver is used for patients with no suspected spinal injury. Both the mouth-to-mouth and mouth-to-nose procedures are no longer accepted as safe for EMR personnel.

53. B: Abdominal thrusts are the most effective method of clearing the airway of an adult or child who is choking; if the patient is large or the EMR is small in size, abdominal thrusts may be given by straddling the patient's legs. Abdominal thrusts are not recommended for infants under 1 year of age or for obese or pregnant patients; in the case of pregnant women or obese patients, chest thrusts may be used instead.

54. D: An OPA should only be used to maintain the airway of unresponsive patients who do not have a gag reflex. The OPA does not maintain an open airway position by itself; thus, the EMR must still manually maintain the patient's airway when using an OPA. The NPA is preferred for patients who are not completely unresponsive or who have a gag reflex. The OPA, NPA, and BVM may be used together.

55. C: The nasopharyngeal airway is preferred for patient who are not completely unresponsive or who have a gag reflex. NPAs are designed to fit infants, children, and adults. NPAs do not have to be removed if the patient becomes responsive. An NPA is contraindicated in patients with skull or facial fractures because it may enter the cranial cavity, causing damage to the brain.

56. A: The patient's little finger is approximately the same size as his or her nostril opening and may be used to select an airway that is approximately the same diameter.

57. C: The airway should never be forced into the nostril. If the NPA will not advance into the nostril, the EMR should attempt to insert it into the opposite nostril; if the airway still does not fit, another airway that is smaller in diameter should be used. Most NPAs are made with the bevel to the left; snipping the end of the airway with scissors will change the bevel from left to right. Petroleum jelly or other non-water–based lubricants should not be used to lubricate the outside of the tube.

58. B: Many elderly patients have thin, easily damaged mucosa or are taking blood-thinning medications such as Coumadin and are thus more prone to nosebleeds; care should be taken when placing an NPA in these patients. It is recommended that the NPA be inserted before placing a BVM. The BVM may be used to ventilate patients with inadequate respirations such as those with a drug overdose; it also acts as an effective infection-control barrier between the EMR and the patient.

59. D: Suctioning is used to remove fluids and other matter from the airway; however, it also removes oxygen. Suctioning should be performed for no more than 15 seconds in adults, 10 seconds in children, and 5 seconds in infants. Before inserting the catheter, fluid and other matter may be removed from the oral cavity by using finger sweeps with a gloved hand. The tip of the catheter should not be placed directly over the back of the tongue, as this may stimulate the gag reflex.

60. C: The MOI should be assessed in trauma patients, or those who have a physical injury caused by an external force. In unresponsive medical patients, or those who have an illness or who have not suffered a physical injury, the family or bystanders should be interviewed to determine the NOI.

61. D: In the scene size-up of a medical patient, the EMR should take the appropriate BSI precautions, determine if the scene is safe, and evaluate the NOI; the need for spinal immobilization should be considered in the scene size-up of trauma patients.

62. C: The ABCs of emergency care are used in the initial assessment of the patient to identify any life-threatening problems in three major areas: Airway, Breathing, and Circulation.

63. C: The AVPU scale is used to assess the patient's mental status; the components of the scale are: Alert, Verbal, Painful, and Unresponsive. The verbal component means that the patient has responded to a loud verbal stimulus. A patient does not necessarily have to initiate a conversation or answer questions to be considered responsive; he or she may simply grunt or groan or look at the EMR in response to a question.

64. D: Because infants and small children have faster breathing and pulse rates than adults, the brachial pulse is taken at the brachial artery in the upper arm and not at the neck or wrist.

65. B: In assessing the mental status of an infant, the EMR should talk to him or her and flick the bottom of the feet. In opening an infant's airway, the head should be in a neutral position and not tilted back as in an adult. In infants and children, the brachial pulse should be obtained at the upper arm and not at the wrist or neck. Because children can maintain a near-normal pulse until almost half of their total blood volume has been depleted, blood pressure is not a reliable indicator of a child's circulation.

66. D: Priority dispatching of EMS involves determining whether basic life support or advanced life support is needed, as well as what response mode should be used; cold response mode, or no lights or siren, or hot response mode, or lights and siren. A focused history and physical examination are conducted after the initial assessment; if the patient has a life-threatening condition, there may not be enough time to perform these steps.

67. B: In assessing a patient, subjective findings are symptoms reported by the patient, family members of the patient, or bystanders, including chest pain, dizziness, and nausea. Objective findings refer to signs, or what the EMR sees, hears, feels, or smells when examining the patient; signs include cool clammy skin or unequal pupils.

68. C: The patient history can be obtained while performing the physical examination or while treating a bleeding wound; there is no need to wait to take vital signs until after the history has been obtained. When obtaining the patient history, the term "drugs" or "recreational drugs" should not be used because they imply abuse; some patients may believe the EMR is attempting to obtain criminal evidence and become uneasy.

69. A: The acronym SAMPLE is used by an EMR to recall the type of questions that should be asked during a patient interview: Signs/symptoms; Allergies; Medications; Pertinent past medical history; Last oral intake; and Events leading to the illness or injury. It is not necessary to know more than the general age of an adult patient; however, a child's age should be obtained to determine what type of treatment should be provided and an adolescent's to determine whether he or she is a minor.

70. C: A rapid, weak pulse may indicate shock, blood loss, a heat or diabetic emergency, or a failing circulatory system, whereas a rapid, strong pulse is associated with high blood pressure, internal bleeding, and fever; a slow, strong pulse is associated with stroke or brain injury. No pulse is indicative of cardiac arrest.

71. B: A rapid, strong pulse is associated with internal bleeding and high blood pressure, while a rapid, weak pulse is associated with shock; however, both a rapid, strong pulse and a rapid, weak pulse are associated with heat emergency. A slow, strong pulse indicates stroke or brain injury.

72. C: A radial pulse may be undetectable if the patient's blood pressure is too low or if an extremity injury is present that blocks blood flow to the distal arm. Because the thumb has its own pulse, it may be mistaken for the patient's pulse and thus should not be used. The absence of a radial pulse alone is not sufficient cause to start CPR.

73. A: Snoring is most often associated with stroke, fractured skull, drug or alcohol abuse, or partial airway obstruction. Wheezing is associated with asthma and rapid, shallow breathing with pneumonia. Patients with a fractured rib may cough blood.

74. B: Skin color, temperature, and moisture may be assessed at the patient's forehead; however, if this is not possible, the abdomen may serve as an alternate site. In some jurisdictions, the extremities may be used as an alternative.

75. B: A cyanotic or bluish skin color may indicate inadequate breathing or heart function; pale skin color may indicate shock, decreased blood pressure, or emotional distress and facial flushing high blood pressure or emotional excitement.

76. C: Jaundiced or yellowish skin color is a sign of liver abnormalities. Cherry red skin indicates the late stages of carbon monoxide poisoning; shock may be indicated by blotchiness or pale skin color.

77. D: Skin that is both cool and moist is usually a sign of anxiety; hot, moist skin may indicate high fever or heat emergency. Goose bumps are associated with chills, communicable disease, or exposure to cold, pain, or fear. Cold, dry skin indicates exposure to cold or diabetic emergency.

78. B: Unequal pupils may indicate stroke or head injury; dilated, nonreactive pupils may indicate shock or reaction to certain medications and constricted, nonreactive pupils central nervous system damage.

79. C: The acronym BP-DOC is used to recall what to look for in a physical exam; B stands for Bleeding; P for Pain; D for Deformities; O for Open wounds; and C for Crepitus, or a grating noise or sensation resulting from broken bone ends rubbing together.

80. D: The acronym DCAP-BTLS is used to recall what to look for during a physical exam; D stands for Deformities; C for Contusions; A for Abrasions; P for Punctures and penetrations; B for Burns; T for Tenderness; L for Lacerations; and S for Swelling.

81. B: The dorsalis pedis pulse is a distal pulse located lateral to the large tendon of the big toe.

82. A: The posterior tibial pulse is a distal pulse that may be taken behind the medial ankle.

83. C: The acronym OPQRST may be used to assess the responsive medical patient and is especially useful when the chief complaint is pain or shortness of breath. O stands for Onset; P for Provocation; Q for Quality; R for Region and radiate; S for Severity; and T for Time.

84. B: The OPQRST mneumonic is used in assessing the responsive medical patient; R stands for region and radiate, indicating where the pain is originating from and to where it is moving or radiating.

85. C: When providing CPR to a child, the rate of compressions is 100/minute, the same as that in adults; the mouth-to-barrier device may be used in both adults and children. When only one rescuer is providing CPR, the rate of compressions to breaths is 30:2 in both children and adults; the depth of compression in children is one third to one half the depth of the chest, compared with 1.5 to 2 inches in adults.

86. D: CPR should not be interrupted for any longer than absolutely necessary; however, if the patient regains a pulse and/or breathing, if another rescuer can take over, or if you are too tired to continue, CPR may be stopped. If the patient has a pulse but is not breathing, continue ventilations at the rate of one breath every 5 to 6 seconds. If the patient has no pulse, continue CPR.

87. C: When arriving on the scene as a lone EMR, you may leave an adult patient alone long enough to call for help; if the patient is a child, 2 minutes of rescue support should be performed before calling for help. If a bystander who is CPR-trained has started CPR, the patient's pulse and breathing should be assessed before taking over; a bystander may be allowed to perform chest compressions while the EMR ventilates the patient.

88. B: When performing two-rescuer CPR, either rescuer may request a change of positions if he or she is tired; however, unless the compressor cannot generate a pulse during compression, the compressor decides when to change positions. The compressor must deliver 30 compressions before switching positions.

89. A: Occasionally, a cracking or popping sound is heard during chest compressions; this is a normal side effect of good chest compression and indicates a separation of the cartilage where the ribs meet the sternum. In adult patients, the ribs may fracture during CPR; however, if this occurs, CPR should not be stopped. The EMR should check his or her hand position, reposition the hands if necessary, and resume CPR.

90. A: CPR should always be provided unless obvious signs of prolonged death such as rigor mortis or pooling of blood are present or if the physician at the scene has accepted responsibility for the patient and has directed you to stop. CPR should be provided even if the patient is terminally ill or very old or if the family has requested you to stop unless a Do Not Resuscitate order has been issued. Even if the patient has been in cardiac arrest for more than 10 minutes, you should not refuse to begin CPR; there are documented cases of patients who have been resuscitated after prolonged periods of time.

91. C: An AED is used to detect abnormal heart rhythms such as ventricular fibrillation and ventricular tachycardia; however, it is not effective in the case of asystole, a condition in which no electrical activity occurs within the heart.

92. B: An AED may be placed on a patient who is over 1 year of age, unresponsive, pulseless, and not breathing.

93. C: Although an AED may be safely placed on a patient lying on a wet surface, it should not be placed if the patient is lying in a pool of water. AEDs should not be placed on patients in a moving vehicle or ambulance or in those with an obstructed airway.

94. A: The defibrillator should be attached immediately; if two EMRs are present, one partner should set up the defibrillator and the other should begin CPR. If the EMR is alone, he or she should attach the defibrillator and call EMS before beginning CPR. Following the shock, the defibrillator will advise you to begin CPR; if the patient goes into a rhythm that is not shockable, the AED will advise you to begin CPR. If the patient does not have a pulse, you should leave the defibrillator attached and continue CPR until more advanced EMS personnel arrive.

95. B: In an adult male, total blood volume is 6.6 liters; a blood loss of 2.2 liters would be considered lethal. In a child, the total blood volume is 1.5 to 2 liters; in an infant, a blood loss of 30 to 50 milliliters would be considered lethal.

96. C: Venous, arterial, and capillary bleeding are all types of external bleeding. In the case of arterial bleeding, blood spurts from an artery with every heart beat and a large amount of blood can be lost in a short amount of time; in venous bleeding, blood flows steadily from a vein and bleeding may be profuse. In patients with capillary bleeding, blood flow is slow.

97. B: In the case of venous bleeding, the color of the blood may appear dark red or deep maroon because it contains little oxygen; in the case of arterial bleeding, the blood is bright red in color. In the case of capillary bleeding, the color of the blood is bright red but not as bright as in arterial bleeding.

98. C: The first step in controlling external bleeding is to apply direct pressure; pressure dressing may also be used; next, elevation with direct pressure should be used, followed by pressure points in the upper arm and groin. A tourniquet should be used only as a last resort.

99. D: Elevation with direct pressure may be used to control bleeding from an arm or leg; it should not be used in patients with suspected fractures or spinal injuries or when objects are impaled in the extremities.

100. C: In the elderly, the survival reflexes present in younger individuals may be blunted due to cardiac disease or medication; thus, the patient's level of consciousness is the most reliable sign of shock due to internal bleeding.

How to Overcome Test Anxiety

Just the thought of taking a test is enough to make most people a little nervous. A test is an important event that can have a long-term impact on your future, so it's important to take it seriously and it's natural to feel anxious about performing well. But just because anxiety is normal, that doesn't mean that it's helpful in test taking, or that you should simply accept it as part of your life. Anxiety can have a variety of effects. These effects can be mild, like making you feel slightly nervous, or severe, like blocking your ability to focus or remember even a simple detail.

If you experience test anxiety—whether severe or mild—it's important to know how to beat it. To discover this, first you need to understand what causes test anxiety.

Causes of Test Anxiety

While we often think of anxiety as an uncontrollable emotional state, it can actually be caused by simple, practical things. One of the most common causes of test anxiety is that a person does not feel adequately prepared for their test. This feeling can be the result of many different issues such as poor study habits or lack of organization, but the most common culprit is time management. Starting to study too late, failing to organize your study time to cover all of the material, or being distracted while you study will mean that you're not well prepared for the test. This may lead to cramming the night before, which will cause you to be physically and mentally exhausted for the test. Poor time management also contributes to feelings of stress, fear, and hopelessness as you realize you are not well prepared but don't know what to do about it.

Other times, test anxiety is not related to your preparation for the test but comes from unresolved fear. This may be a past failure on a test, or poor performance on tests in general. It may come from comparing yourself to others who seem to be performing better or from the stress of living up to expectations. Anxiety may be driven by fears of the future—how failure on this test would affect your educational and career goals. These fears are often completely irrational, but they can still negatively impact your test performance.

> **Review Video:** <u>3 Reasons You Have Test Anxiety</u>
> Visit mometrix.com/academy and enter code: 428468

Elements of Test Anxiety

As mentioned earlier, test anxiety is considered to be an emotional state, but it has physical and mental components as well. Sometimes you may not even realize that you are suffering from test anxiety until you notice the physical symptoms. These can include trembling hands, rapid heartbeat, sweating, nausea, and tense muscles. Extreme anxiety may lead to fainting or vomiting. Obviously, any of these symptoms can have a negative impact on testing. It is important to recognize them as soon as they begin to occur so that you can address the problem before it damages your performance.

> **Review Video: 3 Ways to Tell You Have Test Anxiety**
> Visit mometrix.com/academy and enter code: 927847

The mental components of test anxiety include trouble focusing and inability to remember learned information. During a test, your mind is on high alert, which can help you recall information and stay focused for an extended period of time. However, anxiety interferes with your mind's natural processes, causing you to blank out, even on the questions you know well. The strain of testing during anxiety makes it difficult to stay focused, especially on a test that may take several hours. Extreme anxiety can take a huge mental toll, making it difficult not only to recall test information but even to understand the test questions or pull your thoughts together.

> **Review Video: How Test Anxiety Affects Memory**
> Visit mometrix.com/academy and enter code: 609003

Effects of Test Anxiety

Test anxiety is like a disease—if left untreated, it will get progressively worse. Anxiety leads to poor performance, and this reinforces the feelings of fear and failure, which in turn lead to poor performances on subsequent tests. It can grow from a mild nervousness to a crippling condition. If allowed to progress, test anxiety can have a big impact on your schooling, and consequently on your future.

Test anxiety can spread to other parts of your life. Anxiety on tests can become anxiety in any stressful situation, and blanking on a test can turn into panicking in a job situation. But fortunately, you don't have to let anxiety rule your testing and determine your grades. There are a number of relatively simple steps you can take to move past anxiety and function normally on a test and in the rest of life.

> **Review Video: How Test Anxiety Impacts Your Grades**
> Visit mometrix.com/academy and enter code: 939819

Physical Steps for Beating Test Anxiety

While test anxiety is a serious problem, the good news is that it can be overcome. It doesn't have to control your ability to think and remember information. While it may take time, you can begin taking steps today to beat anxiety.

Just as your first hint that you may be struggling with anxiety comes from the physical symptoms, the first step to treating it is also physical. Rest is crucial for having a clear, strong mind. If you are tired, it is much easier to give in to anxiety. But if you establish good sleep habits, your body and mind will be ready to perform optimally, without the strain of exhaustion. Additionally, sleeping well helps you to retain information better, so you're more likely to recall the answers when you see the test questions.

Getting good sleep means more than going to bed on time. It's important to allow your brain time to relax. Take study breaks from time to time so it doesn't get overworked, and don't study right before bed. Take time to rest your mind before trying to rest your body, or you may find it difficult to fall asleep.

> **Review Video: The Importance of Sleep for Your Brain**
> Visit mometrix.com/academy and enter code: 319338

Along with sleep, other aspects of physical health are important in preparing for a test. Good nutrition is vital for good brain function. Sugary foods and drinks may give a burst of energy but this burst is followed by a crash, both physically and emotionally. Instead, fuel your body with protein and vitamin-rich foods.

Also, drink plenty of water. Dehydration can lead to headaches and exhaustion, especially if your brain is already under stress from the rigors of the test. Particularly if your test is a long one, drink water during the breaks. And if possible, take an energy-boosting snack to eat between sections.

> **Review Video: How Diet Can Affect your Mood**
> Visit mometrix.com/academy and enter code: 624317

Along with sleep and diet, a third important part of physical health is exercise. Maintaining a steady workout schedule is helpful, but even taking 5-minute study breaks to walk can help get your blood pumping faster and clear your head. Exercise also releases endorphins, which contribute to a positive feeling and can help combat test anxiety.

When you nurture your physical health, you are also contributing to your mental health. If your body is healthy, your mind is much more likely to be healthy as well. So take time to rest, nourish your body with healthy food and water, and get moving as much as possible. Taking these physical steps will make you stronger and more able to take the mental steps necessary to overcome test anxiety.

> **Review Video: How to Stay Healthy and Prevent Test Anxiety**
> Visit mometrix.com/academy and enter code: 877894

Mental Steps for Beating Test Anxiety

Working on the mental side of test anxiety can be more challenging, but as with the physical side, there are clear steps you can take to overcome it. As mentioned earlier, test anxiety often stems from lack of preparation, so the obvious solution is to prepare for the test. Effective studying may be the most important weapon you have for beating test anxiety, but you can and should employ several other mental tools to combat fear.

First, boost your confidence by reminding yourself of past success—tests or projects that you aced. If you're putting as much effort into preparing for this test as you did for those, there's no reason you should expect to fail here. Work hard to prepare; then trust your preparation.

Second, surround yourself with encouraging people. It can be helpful to find a study group, but be sure that the people you're around will encourage a positive attitude. If you spend time with others who are anxious or cynical, this will only contribute to your own anxiety. Look for others who are motivated to study hard from a desire to succeed, not from a fear of failure.

Third, reward yourself. A test is physically and mentally tiring, even without anxiety, and it can be helpful to have something to look forward to. Plan an activity following the test, regardless of the outcome, such as going to a movie or getting ice cream.

When you are taking the test, if you find yourself beginning to feel anxious, remind yourself that you know the material. Visualize successfully completing the test. Then take a few deep, relaxing breaths and return to it. Work through the questions carefully but with confidence, knowing that you are capable of succeeding.

Developing a healthy mental approach to test taking will also aid in other areas of life. Test anxiety affects more than just the actual test—it can be damaging to your mental health and even contribute to depression. It's important to beat test anxiety before it becomes a problem for more than testing.

> **Review Video: Test Anxiety and Depression**
> Visit mometrix.com/academy and enter code: 904704

Study Strategy

Being prepared for the test is necessary to combat anxiety, but what does being prepared look like? You may study for hours on end and still not feel prepared. What you need is a strategy for test prep. The next few pages outline our recommended steps to help you plan out and conquer the challenge of preparation.

Step 1: Scope Out the Test

Learn everything you can about the format (multiple choice, essay, etc.) and what will be on the test. Gather any study materials, course outlines, or sample exams that may be available. Not only will this help you to prepare, but knowing what to expect can help to alleviate test anxiety.

Step 2: Map Out the Material

Look through the textbook or study guide and make note of how many chapters or sections it has. Then divide these over the time you have. For example, if a book has 15 chapters and you have five days to study, you need to cover three chapters each day. Even better, if you have the time, leave an extra day at the end for overall review after you have gone through the material in depth.

If time is limited, you may need to prioritize the material. Look through it and make note of which sections you think you already have a good grasp on, and which need review. While you are studying, skim quickly through the familiar sections and take more time on the challenging parts. Write out your plan so you don't get lost as you go. Having a written plan also helps you feel more in control of the study, so anxiety is less likely to arise from feeling overwhelmed at the amount to cover. A sample plan may look like this:

- Day 1: Skim chapters 1–4, study chapter 5 (especially pages 31–33)
- Day 2: Study chapters 6–7, skim chapters 8–9
- Day 3: Skim chapter 10, study chapters 11–12 (especially pages 87–90)
- Day 4: Study chapters 13–15
- Day 5: Overall review (focus most on chapters 5, 6, and 12), take practice test

Step 3: Gather Your Tools

Decide what study method works best for you. Do you prefer to highlight in the book as you study and then go back over the highlighted portions? Or do you type out notes of the important information? Or is it helpful to make flashcards that you can carry with you? Assemble the pens, index cards, highlighters, post-it notes, and any other materials you may need so you won't be distracted by getting up to find things while you study.

If you're having a hard time retaining the information or organizing your notes, experiment with different methods. For example, try color-coding by subject with colored pens, highlighters, or post-it notes. If you learn better by hearing, try recording yourself reading your notes so you can listen while in the car, working out, or simply sitting at your desk. Ask a friend to quiz you from your flashcards, or try teaching someone the material to solidify it in your mind.

Step 4: Create Your Environment

It's important to avoid distractions while you study. This includes both the obvious distractions like visitors and the subtle distractions like an uncomfortable chair (or a too-comfortable couch that makes you want to fall asleep). Set up the best study environment possible: good lighting and a comfortable work area. If background music helps you focus, you may want to turn it on, but otherwise keep the room quiet. If you are using a computer to take notes, be sure you don't have any other windows open, especially applications like social media, games, or anything else that could distract you. Silence your phone and turn off notifications. Be sure to keep water close by so you stay hydrated while you study (but avoid unhealthy drinks and snacks).

Also, take into account the best time of day to study. Are you freshest first thing in the morning? Try to set aside some time then to work through the material. Is your mind clearer in the afternoon or evening? Schedule your study session then. Another method is to study at the same time of day that you will take the test, so that your brain gets used to working on the material at that time and will be ready to focus at test time.

Step 5: Study!

Once you have done all the study preparation, it's time to settle into the actual studying. Sit down, take a few moments to settle your mind so you can focus, and begin to follow your study plan. Don't give in to distractions or let yourself procrastinate. This is your time to prepare so you'll be ready to fearlessly approach the test. Make the most of the time and stay focused.

Of course, you don't want to burn out. If you study too long you may find that you're not retaining the information very well. Take regular study breaks. For example, taking five minutes out of every hour to walk briskly, breathing deeply and swinging your arms, can help your mind stay fresh.

As you get to the end of each chapter or section, it's a good idea to do a quick review. Remind yourself of what you learned and work on any difficult parts. When you feel that you've mastered the material, move on to the next part. At the end of your study session, briefly skim through your notes again.

But while review is helpful, cramming last minute is NOT. If at all possible, work ahead so that you won't need to fit all your study into the last day. Cramming overloads your brain with more information than it can process and retain, and your tired mind may struggle to recall even previously learned information when it is overwhelmed with last-minute study. Also, the urgent nature of cramming and the stress placed on your brain contribute to anxiety. You'll be more likely to go to the test feeling unprepared and having trouble thinking clearly.

So don't cram, and don't stay up late before the test, even just to review your notes at a leisurely pace. Your brain needs rest more than it needs to go over the information again. In fact, plan to finish your studies by noon or early afternoon the day before the test. Give your brain the rest of the day to relax or focus on other things, and get a good night's sleep. Then you will be fresh for the test and better able to recall what you've studied.

Step 6: Take a practice test

Many courses offer sample tests, either online or in the study materials. This is an excellent resource to check whether you have mastered the material, as well as to prepare for the test format and environment.

Check the test format ahead of time: the number of questions, the type (multiple choice, free response, etc.), and the time limit. Then create a plan for working through them. For example, if you have 30 minutes to take a 60-question test, your limit is 30 seconds per question. Spend less time on the questions you know well so that you can take more time on the difficult ones.

If you have time to take several practice tests, take the first one open book, with no time limit. Work through the questions at your own pace and make sure you fully understand them. Gradually work up to taking a test under test conditions: sit at a desk with all study materials put away and set a timer. Pace yourself to make sure you finish the test with time to spare and go back to check your answers if you have time.

After each test, check your answers. On the questions you missed, be sure you understand why you missed them. Did you misread the question (tests can use tricky wording)? Did you forget the information? Or was it something you hadn't learned? Go back and study any shaky areas that the practice tests reveal.

Taking these tests not only helps with your grade, but also aids in combating test anxiety. If you're already used to the test conditions, you're less likely to worry about it, and working through tests until you're scoring well gives you a confidence boost. Go through the practice tests until you feel comfortable, and then you can go into the test knowing that you're ready for it.

Test Tips

On test day, you should be confident, knowing that you've prepared well and are ready to answer the questions. But aside from preparation, there are several test day strategies you can employ to maximize your performance.

First, as stated before, get a good night's sleep the night before the test (and for several nights before that, if possible). Go into the test with a fresh, alert mind rather than staying up late to study.

Try not to change too much about your normal routine on the day of the test. It's important to eat a nutritious breakfast, but if you normally don't eat breakfast at all, consider eating just a protein bar. If you're a coffee drinker, go ahead and have your normal coffee. Just make sure you time it so that the caffeine doesn't wear off right in the middle of your test. Avoid sugary beverages, and drink enough water to stay hydrated but not so much that you need a restroom break 10 minutes into the test. If your test isn't first thing in the morning, consider going for a walk or doing a light workout before the test to get your blood flowing.

Allow yourself enough time to get ready, and leave for the test with plenty of time to spare so you won't have the anxiety of scrambling to arrive in time. Another reason to be early is to select a good seat. It's helpful to sit away from doors and windows, which can be distracting. Find a good seat, get out your supplies, and settle your mind before the test begins.

When the test begins, start by going over the instructions carefully, even if you already know what to expect. Make sure you avoid any careless mistakes by following the directions.

Then begin working through the questions, pacing yourself as you've practiced. If you're not sure on an answer, don't spend too much time on it, and don't let it shake your confidence. Either skip it and come back later, or eliminate as many wrong answers as possible and guess among the remaining ones. Don't dwell on these questions as you continue—put them out of your mind and focus on what lies ahead.

Be sure to read all of the answer choices, even if you're sure the first one is the right answer. Sometimes you'll find a better one if you keep reading. But don't second-guess yourself if you do immediately know the answer. Your gut instinct is usually right. Don't let test anxiety rob you of the information you know.

If you have time at the end of the test (and if the test format allows), go back and review your answers. Be cautious about changing any, since your first instinct tends to be correct, but make sure you didn't misread any of the questions or accidentally mark the wrong answer choice. Look over any you skipped and make an educated guess.

At the end, leave the test feeling confident. You've done your best, so don't waste time worrying about your performance or wishing you could change anything. Instead, celebrate the successful completion of this test. And finally, use this test to learn how to deal with anxiety even better next time.

> **Review Video: 5 Tips to Beat Test Anxiety**
> Visit mometrix.com/academy and enter code: 570656

Important Qualification

Not all anxiety is created equal. If your test anxiety is causing major issues in your life beyond the classroom or testing center, or if you are experiencing troubling physical symptoms related to your anxiety, it may be a sign of a serious physiological or psychological condition. If this sounds like your situation, we strongly encourage you to seek professional help.

Thank You

We at Mometrix would like to extend our heartfelt thanks to you, our friend and patron, for allowing us to play a part in your journey. It is a privilege to serve people from all walks of life who are unified in their commitment to building the best future they can for themselves.

The preparation you devote to these important testing milestones may be the most valuable educational opportunity you have for making a real difference in your life. We encourage you to put your heart into it—that feeling of succeeding, overcoming, and yes, conquering will be well worth the hours you've invested.

We want to hear your story, your struggles and your successes, and if you see any opportunities for us to improve our materials so we can help others even more effectively in the future, please share that with us as well. **The team at Mometrix would be absolutely thrilled to hear from you!** So please, send us an email (support@mometrix.com) and let's stay in touch.

If you'd like some additional help, check out these other resources we offer for your exam:

http://MometrixFlashcards.com/EMT

Additional Bonus Material

Due to our efforts to try to keep this book to a manageable length, we've created a link that will give you access to all of your additional bonus material.

Please visit **https://www.mometrix.com/bonus948/emr** to access the information.